The Silent Thief

Osteoporosis, Exercises and Strategies for Prevention and Treatment

Karine Bohme
with Frances Budden, MD

FIREFLY BOOKS

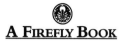

A FIREFLY BOOK

Published by Firefly Books (U.S.) Inc., 2001

U.S. Cataloging-in-Publication Data
  (Library of Congress Standards)

Bohme, Karine.
   The silent thief : osteoporosis, exercises and strategies for prevention and treatment / Karine Bohme with Frances Budden.—1st ed.
[224] p. : ill. ; cm.
Includes bibliographic references and index.
Summary: Exercises and nutritional strategies to help prevent and treat osteoporosis. Includes a comprehensive overview of osteoporosis and drug therapies.
ISBN 1-55297-539-8 (pbk.)
1. Osteoporosis—Prevention. 2. Osteoporosis—Exercise therapy. 3. Osteoporosis—Nutritional aspects. 4. Osteoporosis—Treatment. I. Budden, Frances. II. Title.
 616.716 21 2001 CIP

Published in the United States in 2001 by
Firefly Books (U.S.) Inc.
P.O. Box 1338, Ellicott Station
Buffalo, New York, 14205

Cover illustration: Mark Thurman
Interior design: Gary Beelik
Interior illustrations: Crowle Art
Page layout and cover design: George Walker

Please note:
In the interest of good health, it is always important to consult your doctor before commencing any exercise program, especially if you have a medical condition or are pregnant. All guidelines and warnings should be read carefully. The author and publisher disclaim any liability or loss, personal or otherwise, resulting from the procedures and information in this book.

Printed in Canada

For my husband, Michael, and our new daughter, Annie

Contents

Acknowledgments

I am grateful to the following people, whose expertise, guidance and support helped make this book possible:

Personal trainers Phil Delaire, Shawn Marsland, Anna Lampignano and Tyrone Estabrook for their energy and ideas that inspired much of the exercise section.

Paula Pike, for her invaluable feedback and for buoying my spirits through the writing process.

My private clients—those with osteoporosis and those working towards preventing it—for teaching me more about osteoporosis than any medical textbook could. I am grateful to all my "Ladies and Aunties" who attend my weekly fitness classes and who ask all the right questions. Their continued attendance inspires me to create exciting new ways to keep them kicking for years to come.

Nemit Syriani, office manager at Glendon College, York University, for her unflagging administrative support.

Paula Dunlop whose fearless approach to getting things done helped bring this book to the attention of Pearson Education Canada.

Tracy Bordian, Jennifer Mactaggart and Liba Berry of Pearson Education Canada, without whose editorial support this book would not have been possible.

Dr. Frances Budden, the medical voice of this book, gave energy and expertise to these pages. It has been both a pleasure and an education working with her.

Finally, I am enormously grateful to the family and friends who encouraged and supported me through the writing of this book. To my dear husband, Michael, thank you for your patience and for the wonderful dinners you cooked for me. Your unwavering support helped to make this book a reality.

—*Karine Bohme*

I am indebted to my mentors and patients, who gave me the knowledge to participate in writing this book. The love and support of my husband, Jeffrey, and daughter, Sarah, made it possible for me to research and write my share of the book.

—*Frances Budden*

Introduction

Osteoporosis is the Silent Thief that steals away our bones. It is a degenerative disease that silently weakens bones over time, causing pain, loss of movement, and fractures, and, eventually, seriously affecting quality of life. Osteoporosis is insidious because it frequently goes unnoticed until the sufferer experiences a break or fracture. The disease, in women, often manifests around menopause, and so, with an aging female population the incidence of osteoporosis will rise unless preventative measures are taken. Eighteen million Americans are at risk for osteoporosis and 10 million Americans already have the disease.

If you are a woman between the ages of 50 and 75 and have been diagnosed with osteoporosis, this book is definitely for you. If you are a man or woman of any age, active or not, who is concerned about bone health, this book is also for you. You can *treat* osteoporosis if you have been diagnosed with low bone density, or *prevent* the disease if your bone density is still in the normal range. As with other diseases associated with aging, prevention starts early. Early prevention can help with heart disease, joint stiffness, malnutrition and the symptoms associated with menopause. You can make changes now that will profoundly affect the health of your bones later in life.

How This Book Came About

As a certified personal trainer and fitness instructor, I have spent years designing programs to help my clients improve their levels of fitness. As the baby boomer population ages, the special needs of my clients have increased exponentially. To the many questions I had been asked over the years about exercise and its effect on osteoporosis, my response was typical: "Do weight training and weight-bearing exercises." It wasn't until I was hired by Dr. Frances Budden that I became interested in the relationship between osteoporosis and the positive effects of exercise on the disease.

Dr. Budden was not only my client but is also an osteoporosis specialist at St. Joseph's Health Centre in Toronto. It was a collaboration made in heaven: Dr. Budden has a wealth of information about brittle bones and areas susceptible to osteoporosis. I have the physiological and biomechanical background to design exercises to strengthen those very areas. Dr. Budden referred many of her patients to me, and as my client base grew I became increasingly aware of the need for personal instruction and program design in this area. Wouldn't it be great, I thought, if every person with osteoporosis could have a personal trainer come to his or her home to demonstrate the most effective exercises to treat the disease? Wouldn't it be great if people without osteoporosis could learn and practice the exercises that would help prevent them contracting the disease? And so the idea for this book was born.

How This Book Is Different

Many books about osteoporosis are disease-focused, with minimal practical strategies offered for prevention and treatment. *The Silent Thief* takes a different approach. An exercise-focused book for the prevention and treatment of osteoporosis, it contains strategies *you* can implement to outwit the Silent Thief. Many of these strategies appear here thanks to the invaluable contribution of many knowledgeable and experienced trainers and physicians.

The few osteoporosis books that contain an exercise section focus on nonfunctional exercises that are outdated. They provide only one exercise for even the most susceptible areas and no progressions. *The Silent Thief* teaches the importance of progression by providing a number of exercises, of various intensities, to challenge individuals at all levels. It teaches you that you can actually *enjoy* your fight against osteoporosis.

How This Book Is Organized

The Silent Thief is organized into three parts: Part A provides an overview of osteoporosis from a medical and preventive perspective; Part B contains diet and drug strategies to prevent and treat osteoporosis; and Part C, will help you use exercise to fight the disease.

Chapter 1 gives you the medical perspective on osteoporosis, provides a scientific perspective on bone health and lists the causes and risk factors of osteoporosis.

Chapter 2 focuses on the importance of calcium and Vitamin D in the prevention and treatment of osteoporosis. This chapter explains the roles that these two vital nutrients play in the health of your bones and suggests how to maximize your intake. The information contained here will help you to make dietary and supplemental choices that will mean longer life for your bones.

Chapter 3 discusses other important nutrients that have a positive impact on bone health: magnesium, vitamin K, potassium, phosphorus and boron. Because soy and soy products contain chemicals that mimic the characteristics of estrogen, they play a vital role in skeletal health. This chapter provides you with the best ways to include these substances in your diet.

Chapter 4 presents you with drug-based strategies to prevent and treat osteoporosis, and includes a discussion of the risks and benefits of hormone replacement therapy (HRT).

Chapters 5 to 8 comprise the very heart of the book, as they focus on the positive impact of exercise and functional fitness on bone health. Weight-bearing exercise, resistance training and balance training—the three most effective ways to strengthen bones and prevent falls—are investigated in depth in this section.

Karine Bohme

Not long ago I was weak and sore all over. My husband, Jeffrey, couldn't stand the complaining so he gave me a birthday gift. A personal trainer—Karine! As a result of the exercises she encouraged me to practice, I am no longer sore all over anymore. As a white, 55-year-old, postmenopausal, slight-framed woman, whose mother had a dowager's hump and a fractured hip, I am at high risk for osteoporosis. I learned that exercise and functional fitness are an approach I could take to prevent getting the disease.

I am an internist and a geriatrician with a special interest in osteoporosis. In 1984, I did postgraduate training with the Bone and Mineral Group at the University of Toronto with Doctors Timothy Murray, Joan Harrison and other great and caring physicians. Most of my time was spent at the Metabolic Bone Clinic at St. Michael's Hospital, where I continue to see patients. I am also the director of the Community Osteoporosis Program with Education at St. Joseph's Health Centre, Toronto.

I see the greatest devastation caused by osteoporosis caring for my geriatric patients after they have sustained fractured hips, wrists, arms, legs, backs and pelvises. These fractures cause pain, loss of independence, deformity, disability, reduced quality of life, and in about 20 percent of hip fractures, death. In 1984, our ability to diagnose osteoporosis was primitive and the treatment options were limited. But we've come a long way. In 2001, osteoporosis can be prevented, diagnosed and treated!

The Bone and Joint Decade was officially launched by the United Nations in January 2000 as the decade of global research for preventative and therapeutic initiatives to improve the quality of life for people with osteoporosis, osteoarthritis, rheumatoid arthritis and spinal injuries. This is Karine's and my part toward advancing this initiative.

Frances Budden, MD, FRCPC

PART A

An Overview of the Silent Thief

one

Understanding Osteoporosis

Good health and good sense are two of life's greatest blessings.

— Publius Syrus, 42 BC

Osteoporosis is a systemic skeletal disease characterized by a low **bone mass** and micro-architectural deterioration of the bone with a consequent increase in bone fragility and susceptibility to fracture. In 1993, the Osteoporosis Consensus Development Conference in Hong Kong developed this definition to help us better understand osteoporosis. In other words, osteoporosis is a decrease in bone substance and strength, such that a slight twisting or bending motion, or a trivial fall, will cause a bone to fracture or break. Bones can become so fragile that getting groceries out of the car or bending over to pick up a child will break a bone in your back.

Osteoporosis already affects 10 million Americans, 80% of these are women. Another 12 million women and 10 million men are at risk for osteoporosis. By age 50, one of every four women and one of every eight men has osteoporosis. Moreover, one of every two women and one of every eight men over age 50 will suffer an osteoporosis-related fracture in their lifetime. The National Osteoporosis Foundation estimates that 80 percent of hip fractures occur as a result of osteoporosis. There are about 300,000 hip fractures annually in the United States, with more than one-third of those requiring long-term care, as they can no longer live independently. It is estimated that by 2041 the number of fractured hips will increase to 90,000 annually. If osteoporosis is treated, the expected number of fractures would decrease by 50 percent. Fractures caused by osteoporosis are very costly to the individual, family and society. In 1995, osteoporosis-related hip fractures cost an estimated $13.8 billion.[1]

All About Bones

Bone health is described by three words: normal, **osteopenia**, or **osteoporosis**. In Latin, *osteopenia* means "thin bone" and *osteoporosis* means "porous bone." The difference between osteopenia and osteoporosis is in the degree of bone thinness and weakness. Osteopenic bones are thin and weak, while osteoporotic bones are even thinner and more fragile. Bone mass is measured by a **bone mineral density test** (BMD) and is used to diagnose osteoporosis. This test is also referred to as a **bone density** test or dual energy X-ray absorptiometry (DXA). (See page 18 for more on bone density testing.)

It's a Bone's Life—I

Bones move, support, protect and store. They enable us to move using an intricate system of joints, ligaments, tendons and muscles. Where bones surround structures, such as the brain, heart, lungs and other organs, they provide considerable protection. The interior of the bones is used to house and protect the bone marrow in which blood cells develop. Moreover, the bones are an immense storehouse for **calcium** and other minerals.[2] Bone is a growing, living, ever-changing tissue.

Bones start to form about the third week after conception in the mesoderm, which is one of the early layers in the embryo. By the fourth month of the baby's development in the womb, the skeleton divides into bones for different uses. The axial skeleton consists of the vertebral column (the backbone), the ribs, and the sternum (the breast bone). The shoulders and arms, pelvis and legs make up the appendicular skeleton. The skull and the mandible and maxilla (the jaw bones) develop around the brain. From this beginning, each bone goes on to have a very long and useful life.

Peak Bone Mass

As mentioned earlier, bones start to grow in utero, and continue to grow until we reach adulthood. **Peak bone mass** is the maximum bone density and strength that a person can attain in life. It is the most bone we will ever have during our lives, and this level is reached between the ages of 20 and 30.

The genetic and ethnic differences in bone mass are considerable. If you have a petite mother with osteoporosis, you have a huge chance of having osteoporotic bones. Caucasians and Asians are at a significantly higher risk of developing osteoporosis than African-Americans. But 10% of African-American women over 50 have osteoporosis.

There is little we can do about our genes and ethnicity, but there are many things that we can do to maximize the peak bone mass of children, teens and young adults. Nutrition plays a significant role in attaining peak bone mass (see Chapters 2 and 3). Good basic nutrition, following the *Dietary Guidelines for Americans* (see pages 50–51), is essential for attaining peak bone mass. An active, healthy lifestyle, drinking alcohol in moderation and not smoking all contribute to the attainment of peak bone mass.

Factors Affecting Peak Bone Mass

- Genetics (race, ethnicity, family history)
- Nutrition (calcium, **vitamin D** and healthy eating)
- Exercise
- Lifestyle (drinking alcohol in moderation and not smoking)
- Hormonal factors (age of puberty, **amenorrhea** [absence or abnormal stopping of menstruation])[3]

Do you know the recommended limits for low-risk drinking?

- Not more than two standard* drinks a day
- For a woman, no more than nine drinks a week
- For a man, no more than 14 drinks a week

* A standard drink is defined as 1 bottle of beer, one 6-ounce glass of wine or one 1½ ounce shot of liquor.[4]

Losing Bone

We cannot halt the aging process. The aging of our bones starts in our mid-thirties and continues until we are very old. **Age-related bone loss** is caused by an imbalance between the formation (building) and resorption (taking away) of bone, leading to bone loss and, in some people, osteopenia and osteoporosis. The bones of both men and women are affected by age-related bone loss. Although all of us lose some bone as we age, the rate of loss varies from person to person. Not every older person has osteoporosis, but studies indicate that 15 percent of women in their fifties are osteoporotic, while 50 percent of women in their eighties have osteoporosis.[5] In women, the hormone **estrogen** plays a significant role in maintaining bone health by preventing bone loss. At **menopause**, lack of estrogen causes rapid bone loss, particularly for the first ten years after menopause, leading to **postmenopausal osteoporosis**. Women experience the effects of both aging and menopause in bone loss, while in men only the effect of aging causes loss of bone.

Broken bones or fractures arise as a result of thin, fragile, osteoporotic bones. Osteoporosis and fractures are a major health problem, causing pain and reduced physical function, independence and self-esteem. Common sites of fracture are the back bones or vertebrae, wrist, and hip, which is the most serious. Two general factors determine whether an individual will eventually develop osteoporosis: peak bone mass and the rate of bone loss. Assuming that two women lose bone at the same yearly rate beginning at age 50, the woman with the least bone will become osteoporotic sooner and be more likely to break a bone at an earlier age. Conversely, if two women have an

NORMAL BONE   **OSTEOPOROTIC BONE**

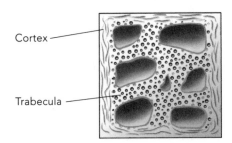 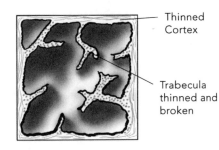

Cortex

Trabecula

Thinned Cortex

Trabecula thinned and broken

identical amount of bone, the woman with the more rapid rate of bone loss will be at risk of fracture sooner. Both low bone mass and a rapid rate of bone loss at menopause are risk factors for future fractures.

The Science of the Silent Thief

Through science and research, osteoporosis is better understood and, as a result, several methods for prevention and treatment of the disease have been discovered. First, let's talk about the genetics of bone, bone cells and the structure of bone.

Genetics of Bone

Osteoporosis has a strong genetic component. It is intuitive to all of us that if a tiny 85-year-old woman with a hip fracture has a petite 50-year-old daughter, the daughter is at high risk for osteoporosis. However, intuition isn't good science. A tremendous amount of research is being done to turn this intuition into science, which will become treatments and cures for osteoporosis. In one example of exciting new research, scientists have found that our genes cause primitive cells in the bone to change into either fat cells or osteoblasts (bone-building cells). As we age, more fat cells are formed, thus less bone. Scientists are searching for a mechanism to stop the fat cells from forming, which would make more bone cells and subsequently more bone.[6] In the future, this research may result in finding a treatment for osteoporosis. Another research initiative has found a gene that regulates vitamin D metabolism. **Vitamin D** is the vitamin that the body makes with the aid of the ultraviolet rays from sunshine on the skin. Vitamin D enables the body to efficiently absorb calcium from the food that is eaten. Some people with osteoporosis don't have this gene, which makes their calcium absorption inefficient.[7]

Bone Cells

There are three main types of cells in bones: **osteoblasts**, **osteoclasts** and **osteocytes**, which are active in making and maintaining bone. The osteoblast builds bone, in a process known as **formation**. The osteoclast chews, removes or destroys bone, which is called **resorption**. Remember, blasts build and clasts chew! This process of continual resorption and formation is called **remodeling**. The osteocyte is an osteoblast that has finished its job of active bone building and has settled down in mature bone. The osteocyte forms a connecting network in mature bone, responding to the work that the bones are being asked to do and sending signals through the bone. When a joint is moved to a different position, the muscles and ligaments either push or pull on the bones. This process is called **mechanical loading**. The bone's internal structure is arranged so as to resist all such forces.

How do bones renew themselves? Osteoblasts turn on a pre-osteoclast or a baby osteoclast, which changes to an up-and-running osteoclast. Osteoclasts are remarkable cells that perform a huge job: they are the "demolition crew" that removes old bone in preparation for its replacement with new bone. To begin this process, the inside of the osteoclast becomes acid, and signals go back and forth from the osteoclast to the bone. The osteoclast settles on an area of bone that needs renovation or remodeling, then seals off the area where it will work so that the acids don't leak out and destroy bone that is new and healthy. The edge of the osteoclast that is against the bone to be destroyed becomes ruffled to give a larger working surface, and the chewing up of old bone begins. Once the osteoclast has removed all of the old bone, the osteoblast moves in and forms **osteoid**, a protein-containing material, in the hole that the osteoclast has made. Osteoid is a soft framework that becomes calcified (or hardened) with calcium and forms a strong, new healthy bone material called calcium hydroxyapatite. This combination of protein and calcium makes bone strong, yet flexible enough to withstand stress or heavy loads.

Structure of Bone

Osteoclasts and osteoblasts do not function randomly or without purpose. In the cortex (the hard, strong outer shell of a bone), they work within hollow microscopic tubes that allow the blood vessels access to the bone. These tubes resist bending so that the outer shell of a bone is very strong, and they bind together so that a bone is one continuous structure in which osteocytes are embedded; the osteoctyes send messages through the bone when there is mechanical loading. In trabecular bone, which is the internal supporting structure or struts of the bone, the osteoclasts and osteoblasts work on an extremely small, flat surface, forming layer upon layer of new bone.[8]

It's a Bone's Life—2

Bone cells don't live forever: they do their job, and then they die. This dying of the cells seems to be programmed specifically for each cell type. Preplanned or programmed cell death is called **apoptosis**. In osteoporosis, apoptosis of the osteoblast (the bone builder) is increased, leaving fewer osteoblasts to do their building job. Bones are very active metabolically as remodeling is a non-stop process: children get a whole new skeleton every two years; healthy, young adults get a whole new skeleton every seven to ten years. Yes, the whole skeleton changes over.

As we age, the ability to form new bone and take away old bone slows to the point where in very old, osteoporotic bones it can take up to 12 years to remodel the skeleton. From birth to 20 years of age, bone building occurs at a rate faster than bone chewing or destroying, so that by age 20 bones are larger, heavier and denser. From age 20 to 35 or so, the rates of building bone and destroying bone are equal. From 35 onwards, bone is built more slowly than it is destroyed. Aging causes a continuous slowing of the remodeling process, such that bone is being destroyed more quickly than it is being built. At menopause, this process of destruction is accelerated by loss of estrogen, which turns off the osteoclasts. Once estrogen is lost, the osteoclasts seem to go crazy, chewing up the bone.[9]

Up to one-third of your body's bone is replaced each year by the process of remodeling. This means that one-third of your skeleton is less than one year old.

What Promotes Remodeling?

The shape and structure of any bone are adapted to its function and to the stresses and strains on the bone. As explained previously, bones alter their shape and structure by remodeling. During its growth period and in adult life, each bone is continually being modified to maintain its function against changes in the stresses upon it.

The cortex (hard outer layer of bone) makes up 70 to 80 percent of the skeleton. The inside of a bone is made up of struts, or trabecullae, which support the bone. The skeleton consists of 20 to 30 percent **trabecular bone**. These trabecullae run in directions suited to the function of a specific bone. For example, a vertebra or a back bone has an outside hard layer (the cortex) and inside, trabecullae or struts that are oriented vertically and horizontally. If an osteoporotic strut gets thinner and thinner, it will eventually break. When one strut breaks, it causes the other nearby struts to become fatigued or weakened as they have to work harder. Fatiguing causes further damage to the bone and leads to fracturing or breaking of the other struts and further fracturing. If enough struts break, the cortex has no support and it collapses, leaving a broken or fractured vertebra. Vertebrae fracture spontaneously, while other bones (such as the wrist, hip and upper arm bone) usually fracture because of a fall, however trivial the fall may be.

Osteoporosis: Are You at Risk?

Some people are more likely to get osteoporosis than others. The more risk factors you have, the greater the risk. In addition to low bone mineral density and low peak bone mass, the risk factors include:

- personal history of fracture as an adult
- history of fracture in a first-degree relative
- current cigarette smoking
- low body weight (under 127 pounds)
- advanced age
- Caucasians carry the greatest risk, but people from all ethnic groups suffer from osteoporosis
- dementia
- female sex
- estrogen deficiency
- early menopause (before age 45)
- surgical removal of both ovaries
- prolonged premenopausal amenorrhea (the absence of regular menstrual cycles for longer than one year)
- low testosterone levels in men
- a lifelong history of calcium deficiency and low levels of vitamin D
- alcoholism
- impaired eyesight despite adequate correction
- a repeated history of falls
- inadequate physical activity

○ use of certain medications (steroids, anticonvulsants, excessive thryoid hormone, certain cancer treatments, heparin therapy)

Reprinted with permission from "How Strong Are Your Bones?"
2000 National Osteoporosis Foundation, Washington, DC 20036

It is important to note that people with no risk factors may still develop the disease.[10]

Fractures: Are You at Risk?

As we age, our risk for osteoporosis and fractures increases greatly. Women are at higher risk than men, but men are also at risk. Each year in the United States, 1.5 million people fracture a bone. Caucasian and Asian women suffer from osteoporosis in greater numbers than African-American women due mainly to differences in the amount and strength of bone, as African-Americans appear to have a genetic predisposition to larger bones. The average calcium intake of Asians has been observed to be about half that of Western population groups. Slender body structure with weight under 130 pounds (60 kilograms) also increases the risk for osteoporosis.

If you have had an early menopause (which means that your menstrual periods have stopped) or you have had your ovaries surgically removed before age 45, you are at great risk. The teenage girl or woman who experiences irregular menstrual periods is at very high risk, particularly if her periods have stopped because of over exercising or a physical activity such as ballet dancing, or if she is suffering from an eating disorder like anorexia nervosa. Most adolescents with anorexia fail to develop strong bones during this phase in their growth.

If a family member (particularly a close relative, such as a mother, grandmother, father, sister or aunt) has had osteoporosis or a fracture, you too are at very high risk. Lifestyle also makes a huge difference to bone health. A lifelong low calcium intake, cigarette smoking, heavy alcohol use and a sedentary lifestyle all contribute to bone loss, osteoporosis and fractures.

As mentioned earlier, if you have already sustained one fracture, you are at huge risk of sustaining another one. You are at greater risk of fracturing a wrist, vertebra, hip or other bone if you have a low bone mineral density. A tendency to fall, poor balance, poor vision or dementia puts a person at very high risk for falls and fractures. A previous fracture and a low bone mineral density are the most important and best predictors of a fragility fracture. Other predictors for a fractured hip include, in women: height greater than 66 inches (168 centimeters), weight less than 127 pounds (58 kilograms), a history of smoking and a family history that includes a mother with a hip fracture.

The most common sites for osteoporotic fractures are the wrist, spine and hip.

PREVENTING FALLS

The majority of fractures, except for spontaneous spinal fractures, are caused by falls. Most falls happen to women in their homes in the afternoon. Falls cause fractures of the wrist, upper arm and hip.

Prevent falls by modifying your environment:

Indoors:

- Remove all loose wires, cords and throw rugs from floors. Make sure all other rugs are anchored and smooth.
- Install grab bars, nonskid tape or rubber mats in the bathtub or shower and in the kitchen near the sink and stove. Make sure that all stairways have secure handrails on both sides.
- Make certain that your house is well lit. Turn on lights if you are going out in the evening or if you get up out of bed during the night.
- Wear sturdy, rubber-soled shoes.

Outdoors:

- Repair cracked sidewalks.
- Install handrails on stairs and steps.
- Trim shrubbery along the pathway to your house.
- Install adequate lighting around doorways and along walkways leading to doors.

During winter:

- Exercise indoors at home or at a health club, or walk at a mall. If you live in an apartment, walk up to the top of the building and down, zigzagging from floor to floor.
- Shovel and salt sidewalks to clear snow and ice. Get help if you need it!
- Wear low-heeled footwear with grooved treads.

Prevent falls by modifying your behavior:

- Many falls are caused by medications such as sedatives, and by caffeine, smoking and alcohol, which affect alertness and balance, particularly during the night. Reduce your intake of these substances.
- Poor vision or hearing, impaired muscle strength and diseases that affect balance, coordination or reflexes also lead to falls. See Chapters 7 and 8 for exercises that will help you to improve your balance.
- Maintain your body weight by eating a healthy amount of nutritious food (see Chapters 2 and 3).

If you are at risk for falls or have had a fall or fracture, seriously consider hip padding to prevent a devastating hip fracture. You can get free information about this at: **www.hipsaver.com** on the Web (telephone 1-800-358-4477 toll-free or 1-781-828-3880); or **www.safehip.com** (telephone 1-877-728-3447 toll-free or 1-781-828-3880). And remember—if you fall, bring it to the attention of your doctor immediately.

Acute Vertebral Fractures: An Important Note

If you have a sudden onset of acute back pain, you may have an acute fracture of your vertebra. Call your doctor immediately. Don't suffer in silence! Vertebral fractures take 8 to 12 weeks to heal as does any other fracture, but a vertebral fracture can't be put in a cast like a broken arm or leg can. Don't despair; a lot can be done to make you comfortable and get you back on your feet, including the following:

Good Pain Control

Good pain control is really important, as you will feel better and be able to get up sooner. You will also eat and sleep better. Pain is controlled with medications such as acetaminophen, nonsteroidal and anti-inflammatory drugs, COX2 inhibitors and various narcotics, depending on the severity of the pain. Your doctor will assist you with pain control.

Support Garment

A support garment will give support to your back, particularly when you are sitting, walking or riding in a car.

Physiotherapy

Physiotherapy can help with pain relief, as a lot of the pain may be due to muscle spasm. Hot packs, gentle massage and eventually an exercise program designed specifically for your back can be extremely helpful.

Good Nutrition

Good general nutrition provides adequate calories so that you don't lose weight, adequate protein so that you don't lose muscle mass and adequate fruits and vegetables so that you are ensured of continued health and vigor.

Calcium and Vitamin D Supplements

If you have not already been on calcium and vitamin D supplements, it is time to start.

If you have had one fracture, you have a 20 percent chance of having another fracture within a year. So do what you can to prevent further falls and fractures (see pages 14–15).

If you have back pain and think you have a fracture, go to your doctor. Don't take a vertebral fracture lying down!

Many digestive tract conditions interfere with the body's ability to absorb calcium and other nutrients essential for healthy bone.

Men and Osteoporosis

Osteoporosis is not exclusive to women. Unlike women, however, men rarely get osteoporosis in middle age. Rather, they become osteoporotic and start to fracture at an older age, at about 70. If men over age 60 have a spine X-ray, 10 percent are found to have vertebral fractures. Men who are tall (over 72 inches [184 centimeters]) or underweight (under 142 pounds [65 kilograms]) are more likely to be osteoporotic. Moreover, a low level of male sex hormone (testosterone) may cause osteoporosis. Many risk factors are similar for men and women, such as advancing age, cigarette smoking, heavy alcohol use and an inactive lifestyle.

Osteoporosis is not an "old lady's disease." Women in their teens, twenties and thirties can get osteoporosis, too. The diets of body-conscious teens often lack calcium-rich milk and milk products. Including these foods in your diet from a very young age optimizes the strength and health of your bones. Remember that prevention of osteoporosis starts early.

Detecting the Silent Thief

The best way to determine if you have osteoporosis is to have a bone mineral density test. The more risk factors you have, the greater your risk of developing or having osteoporosis. Besides the risk factors discussed earlier, consider the following in your decision to be assessed for osteoporosis:

1. You have completed an osteoporosis risk checklist and you think you are at risk.

2. You experience back pain. Back pain is caused by many problems, osteoporosis being only one. The back pain of osteoporosis can start suddenly from an acutely fractured backbone, or it can be a chronic, aching, burning pain, usually between the shoulder blades or in the lower back.

3. You are getting shorter. Your family tells you that you are shrinking. You have noticed that your clothes don't fit well and your tummy is sticking out. You are getting a **dowager's hump** (a hump in the upper back). The dowager's hump (also known as **kyphosis**) is associated with height loss, which means that the bones in your back have already started to fracture. By age 65, about one inch of height is normally lost due to the normal aging process, caused by a decreased amount of water in the disks (the little cushions between each vertebra or back bone). If you have lost more than one inch in height, you need a bone mineral density test to assess your bone health.

4. You are a woman who has had a fracture after age 40.

If you are at risk or have back pain, height loss or a fracture after age 40, ask your doctor for a bone mineral density test.

Bone Mineral Density Test

The bone mineral density test measures amount of bone mass (bone mineral content or BMC) and how tightly the bone is packed (bone mineral density or BMD). In other words, the bone mineral density test measures the amount of calcium in your bones. Your BMD is compared to normal groups: "age-matched," which compares your BMD to someone of your age and with your body size, and "young, normal," which compares your BMD to the peak density of healthy young adults. The difference between your BMD and that of a healthy, young adult is described as a **standard deviation** (SD), a measure of how far a person is from the "normal, healthy, young adult" value. Usually, one SD below zero equals a 10 to 12 percent decrease in bone density.

The World Health Organization provides the following definitions to help diagnose osteoporosis:

- **Normal:** BMD falls within one SD of a "young, normal" adult
- **Low bone mass or osteopenia:** BMD falls one to 2.5 SD below that of "young, normal" adult
- **Osteoporosis:** BMD falls 2.5 SD below that of a "young, normal" adult
- **Severe osteoporosis:** BMD falls below 2.5 SD with one or more fragility fractures[10]

The most commonly used BMD test is a dual energy X-ray absorptiometry (DXA). This test measures the bone density of the spine at the first to the fourth lumbar vertebrae, which are just above and below your waist level, and of either the right or left hip. The test takes 5 to 20 minutes and is painless, with very low radiation exposure. A routine chest X-ray exposes a person to 100 to 150 microsieverts of radiation, while a DXA exposes you to only 1 to 5 microsieverts. (A microsievert is a measurement for radiation exposure.) An X-ray of the spine detects osteoporosis only after 25 to 30 percent of the bone has been lost, but it does detect fractures of the vertebrae, osteoarthritis and other common causes of back pain. An X-ray of the spine is useful to diagnose osteoporosis where a bone mineral density test is not available.

A bone mineral density test functions in a number of ways. It can: detect osteoporosis before a fracture occurs; predict your chances of having a fracture; assess the rate of bone loss with repeated measurements; and monitor the effectiveness of drug treatment for osteoporosis.

Always remember to have your repeat bone mineral density tests done on the same machine at about the same time of year. Each bone density machine is slightly different from another. Your bone density fluctuates with the seasons; it's slightly higher in the summer and lower in the winter.

Currently, experts don't recommend bone mineral density testing for all women, as it is not a screening tool but the best way to rule out or confirm the diagnosis of osteoporosis. The decision to do a bone mineral density test should be made by you and your doctor based on your risk factors. It has been suggested that a BMD test should be done on:

- All postmenopausal women under age 65 who have one or more risk factors for osteoporosis besides menopause
- All women age 65 and older regardless of additional risk factors
- Postmenopausal women and older men with a fracture
- Women who are considering therapy for osteoporosis, if a BMD would facilitate the decision

Once the bone mineral density test is done and you know if your bones are normal, osteopenic or osteoporotic, then you and your family doctor can decide who will manage and treat your bones. Many family doctors and specialists are experts in osteoporosis, including:

- Endocrinologists, specialists in disorders of the glands, for example, thyroid disease and diabetes
- Geriatricians, specialists in the problems and diseases of aging
- Gynecologists, specialists in the diseases of women's reproductive systems
- Orthopedic surgeons, specialists in the preservation and restoration of the function of the skeletal system
- Rheumatologists, specialists in the diseases of the joints and related structures

Some hospitals have multidisciplinary osteoporosis programs, which provide teaching from a dietitian, pharmacist and physiotherapist, as well as medical care. Your own doctor may be the best person to treat you, as she or he knows your medical history, lifestyle and special needs.

If you find out that you have osteopenia or osteoporosis, your doctor will take a history and do a physical examination. You will be asked many questions to determine that you do not have secondary osteoporosis, which is osteoporosis caused by any medical problem other than aging and menopause. The most common causes of secondary osteoporosis are:

- Malnutrition
- Vitamin D deficiency, called osteomalacia
- Endocrine diseases: hyperparathyroidism; hyperthyroidism; excess glucocorticoids; diabetes mellitus
- Drugs—anticonvulsants; steroids
- Severe heart, lung, liver or kidney disease
- Some blood diseases, such as thalassemia
- Some cancers, such as lymphoma, leukemia and multiple myeloma
- Rheumatoid arthritis

Certain chronic diseases, such as congestive heart failure, chronic lung disease and diabetes, seem to put people at greater risk for osteoporosis. It is important to diagnose these diseases so that they can be properly investigated and treated. After appropriate treatment of the disease, the osteoporosis caused by the disease can then be treated.

Specific blood tests are done to exclude other causes of osteoporosis besides aging and menopause. Some of these tests are complete blood count, serum calcium, serum albumin, alkaline phosphatase, serum creatinine, and serum protein electrophoresis. All of these tests should be normal in osteoporosis, except that alkaline phosphatase may be slightly elevated if there has been a recent fracture. Other more specialized tests can be done if necessary to check vitamin D and parathyroid hormone levels.

Special Blood and Urine Tests

Bone remodeling results in byproducts—bits and pieces of the molecules that make up bone—in the blood and urine. These byproducts of bone metabolism are called biochemical or bone markers. Blood and urine tests can detect these markers and give information about the rate of bone remodeling. These tests determine if you are losing bone at a rate that is faster than normal, and can also monitor your response to drug therapy for osteoporosis. However, they do not diagnose osteoporosis and are not a substitute for bone mineral density testing. Remember—osteoblasts build or form bone and osteoclasts chew or remove bone. Bone-specific alkaline phosphatase is the bone marker in blood for osteoblast activity. The marker for osteoclast activity, **NTx** [N-teleopeptide cross links] is found in blood or urine, but is more commonly tested in urine.

Another test that is sometimes done to rule out other problems is a **bone scan**. A bone scan is different from a bone mineral density (BMD) test in that it is not used to diagnose osteoporosis. To perform a bone scan, the physician injects a dye that allows a scanner to see "hot spots," which might be fractures, arthritis, cancer in the bone or other lesions. A bone biopsy, in which the physician uses a special needle to take a small bone sample from the hip, is very occasionally done to rule out osteomalacia, a bone disease that shares symptoms with osteoporosis but which is due to vitamin D deficiency.

The Bare Bones

- Osteoporosis affects 10 million Americans, and by age 50, one of every four women and one of every eight men has osteoporosis.

- Bone health is described by three words: normal, osteopenia or osteoporosis, based on bone mass or the amount of bone present. Bone mass is measured by a bone mineral density (BMD) test.

- Broken bones or fractures occur as a result of thin, fragile, osteoporotic bones. Common sites of fracture are the spine, wrist and hip.

- The three main types of cells in bones are osteoblasts, osteoclasts and octeocytes. Osteoblasts build bone; osteoclasts chew and clear bone; osteocytes form a connecting network in mature bone. The whole process is called remodeling.

- Most fractures are caused by falls. Prevent falls by modifying your environment: remove all loose wires, cords and throw rugs, install grab bars and rubber mats in the bathroom, light your house well and wear sturdy, rubber-soled shoes. Take special care outside during the winter months.

- Men do become osteoporotic and start to fracture at an older age than women, at about 70. A low level of male sex hormone, called testosterone, may cause osteoporosis in men.

Outwitting the Silent Thief through Prevention and Treatment

Two

The Bone Boosters:
Calcium and Vitamin D

The best method of preventing osteoporosis is to ensure optimal bone growth and preservation of bone as life progresses.

—Jens Dirderich Ringe, *Calcium and Health*

Calcium: A Bone's Best Friend

We cannot live without calcium. It is, in fact, the most abundant mineral in the body. As adults, we have 2.5 pounds (one kilogram) or more of calcium in our bodies. While its role in bone is extremely important, calcium performs an array of vital functions elsewhere in the body. Ninety-nine percent of the body's calcium is present in the bones, while one percent is present in the cells or circulating in the blood. Besides providing strength for bones, calcium is also important to: the regulation of muscle contraction; the clotting of blood; the transmission of nerve impulses; the secretion of hormones; and the activation of enzyme reactions.

Regulating Blood Calcium

Bone is living and changing tissue that can exchange calcium with the blood at any time. Blood calcium refers to the level of calcium in the blood, which is carefully controlled by the body so that its concentration in the blood will remain constant at all times. Because 99 percent of the body's calcium occurs in the bones, our skeleton serves as a calcium bank that offers a ready supply of the mineral should our blood calcium level drop.

Blood calcium is vital to many physiological processes and its concentration is closely regulated. The control regulators are a system of hormones and vitamin D. The hormones include **calcitonin** (made by the thyroid gland) and **parathyroid hormone** (made by the parathyroid gland). When calcium is abundant in the blood, the thyroid gland releases calcitonin, which causes the osteoblasts to build new bone using calcium from the blood. When blood calcium is low, the parathyroid glands release parathyroid hormone, which works with vitamin D to affect three organ systems. First, vitamin D speeds up calcium absorption from the intestine into the blood; second, both vitamin D and parathyroid hormone promote calcium to be reabsorbed in the kidney; and third, both parathyroid hormone and vitamin D stimulate osteoclasts to clear away bone and release calcium into the blood.

As you see, the calcium in bone provides a nearly inexhaustible source of calcium for the blood and cells. For optimal health, blood calcium levels must remain constant. If you starve the body of calcium, you starve the bones.

Calcium Absorption

Calcium intake and **calcium absorption** are two different things. You can consume large amounts of calcium through diet or through supplements without the substance ever reaching the bones. The body's ability to absorb calcium is helped and hindered by many factors. Calcium absorption is aided by stomach acid because it makes the mineral soluble (able to mix and dissolve). **Lactose** (the sugar in milk) helps in calcium absorption in the intestine. Like lactose, vitamin D causes calcium to be absorbed in the intestine by helping to make a protein that binds calcium. It is no mistake that milk is the product chosen to be fortified with vitamin D.

Only 30 percent of calcium taken into the body is absorbed in adults. Children and pregnant and nursing women absorb 50 percent because more calcium-binding protein is manufactured during these times. With only one-third of the calcium that you take in being absorbed, it is essential to know the factors that maximize calcium absorption so that you can make informed choices about diet and supplementation. The better that calcium is absorbed, the more available it is for use by the body. To know how to optimize calcium absorption in your body, you need to be aware of and avoid overconsumption of substances that hinder absorption: caffeine, sodium, protein and fiber.

Caffeine

A substance that increases fluid loss from the body, caffeine causes calcium to be taken out of the body through the kidney into the urine. One caffeinated beverage can increase calcium excretion up to four hours after it is consumed, removing up to 50 mg of calcium from the body![1] Caffeine is found in coffee, tea and some cola beverages. Consumption of these beverages should be limited to two to three cups a day, provided that your calcium intake is adequate. If you consume more that three cups a day, increase your calcium intake by drinking a glass of milk for every extra cup of tea/cola/coffee you have or by making some of your coffees café lattes.

Sodium

Sodium is a mineral that is essential to healthy functioning because it helps to maintain a proper balance of body fluids. Since salt cannot be made by the body, it must come from the diet. The problem is that too much sodium increases calcium loss in the urine. Many Americans consume too much sodium—about 3000 mg too much each day. Dietician Leslie Beck, RD, suggests that for every 500 mg increase in your sodium intake (about one-fifth of a teaspoon), you must consume an additional 40 mg of calcium to make up for the increased loss. To reduce your sodium intake, avoid using a saltshaker, and keep highly processed foods and salty snacks out of your diet.

Protein

Protein intake needs to be finely balanced. Eating enough protein protects against a low bone mineral density and hip fractures; too much protein in the diet causes the blood to be slightly more acid than ideal, which causes loss of precious calcium in the urine. A recent study found that increasing daily dietary protein by 40 to 80 g above the recommended allowance increased the amount of calcium in the urine by 10 percent a day.[2] As low-carbohydrate/high-protein diets have become popular, excessive protein consumption has become an issue around calcium and bone density.

To calculate your daily protein needs, multiply your body weight in kilograms by the **U.S. Recommended Daily Allowance (RDA).** One pound equals .4536 kilograms. The female RDA for protein is 0.8 g/kg for someone who participates in no regular exercise, and 1.2 g/kg for someone who exercises regularly. So, a 120 lb (55 kg) woman who exercises needs 66 g of protein a day (55 x 1.2 g/kg). Half a cup of tinned salmon, one egg, one ounce of cheddar cheese and two cups of milk in a day would satisfy this requirement.

Fiber

Dietary fiber, once ingested, travels all the way down the digestive system to the large bowel. It speeds the movement of food breakdown products through the bowel. It increases the weight, number, consistency and water content of feces. It binds to cholesterol and salts in bile and aids in bacterial activity in the bowel. For the most part, dietary fiber cannot be broken down by the human digestive system and is passed as waste product. **Soluble fiber** is found in fruit, beans, food gums and oats. **Insoluble fiber** is found in cereals. Generally, soluble fiber is responsible for binding and removing "bad" cholesterol from the body, and insoluble fiber increases fecal bulk and frequency.

A diet high in **phytic acid**, which is found in the bran of whole grains, is likely to interfere with calcium absorption. This acid binds to a variety of minerals, including calcium, to form insoluble salts that are excreted by the body as waste. To decrease phytic acid consumption, try to get more of your fiber from fruits and vegetables rather than from grains.

U.S. Recommended Daily Allowance for fiber is 25–30 g/day. This should be accompanied by adequate water intake. Dietary fiber can be found in brown rice, asparagus, broccoli, celery, carrots, yams, corn, bran, rolled oats and whole wheat.

Boning Up: Calcium Intake Recommendations

Daily calcium intake has recently been increased due to a greater understanding of the role that calcium plays in bone development. See the table below for recommended calcium intakes.

Recommended Daily Calcium Intakes

AGE	INTAKE
Birth – 6 months	400 mg
6 months – 1 year	600 mg
1 – 10	800-1200 mg
11 – 24	1200-1500 mg
25-50 (women and men)	1000 mg
51 – 64 (women on ERT and men)	1000 mg
51+ (women not on ERT)	1500 mg
65 or older	1500 mg
Pregnant or lactating	1200-1500 mg

from the National Institutes of Health

Calcium intake for girls in the 10-to-12 age group should be at the higher end of the range, as on average girls go through their adolescent growth spurt two years earlier than boys. The recommended intake for the 50+ group has also been increased, as the risk of osteoporosis in this group is high. It is important to note that other studies show that individuals can tolerate up to of 2500 mg of calcium daily.

Raising bone-healthy children starts at home. Encourage your children to consume calcium-rich foods. There are a wide variety of foods and drinks that are high in calcium and that appeal to most kids. Chocolate milk, milkshakes, frozen yogurt, cheese pizza and macaroni-and-cheese all contain more than 250 mg of calcium per 100 g serving. What kid wouldn't love these foods?

Dietary Sources of Calcium

A basic North American diet with no milk products contains only 200 to 300 mg of calcium. Black coffee, juice, toast and an egg for breakfast; juice or a soft drink, a tuna sandwich, fruit, and cake for lunch; and meat, potatoes, a vegetable, salad and pie for supper may appear to be a healthy diet, but there is something essential missing—milk products and calcium-rich foods. The more calcium that you get from food sources, the better. The calcium in food sources is more readily absorbed and will offer other important nutrients for overall health. Consult the table below to help you achieve your recommended daily intake of calcium.

Calcium Content of Selected Foods (in milligrams per 100g serving)

Food	Calcium Content	Food	Calcium Content	Food	Calcium Content
Kelp	1093	Milk (non-fat)	120	Dates	59
Cheddar cheese	750	Milk (1%)	120	Prunes (dried)	51
Swiss cheese	660	Wheat bran	119	Pumpkin seeds	51
Milk powder (dry)	315	Milk (whole)	118	Beans (cooked)	50
Collard leaves	250	Sesame seeds	110	Oysters	50
Kale	249	Olives (ripe)	106	Common cabbage	49
Turnip greens	246	Broccoli	103	Soybean sprouts	48
Almonds	234	Parmesan cheese	103	Shrimp	47
Brewer's yeast	210	Cottage cheese	94	Orange	41
Parsley	203	Bok choy	80	Celery	41
Salmon (can w/bones)	202	Bread (whole wheat, 3 slices)	75	Cashews	38
Yogurt	120	Black currants	60	Rye grain	38
Dandelion greens	187	Soybeans (cooked)	73	Carrot	37
Brazil nuts	186	Pecans	73	Barley	34
Goat's milk	129	Wheat germ	72	Cantaloupe (small)	34
Tofu	128	Peanuts	69	Sweet potato	32
Figs (dried)	126	Romaine lettuce	68	Brown rice	32
Buttermilk	121	Apricots (dried)	67	Beef (roasted)	8
Sunflower seeds	120	Raisins	62	Banana	6

> Calcium is best taken with food in doses not greater than 500 or 600 mg, at least three hours apart.

On average, high levels of calcium are found almost exclusively in a single group of foods—milk and milk products (yogurt and cheese). Do you eat 100 g of collard leaves or kale a day? If you do, congratulations, but I'm willing to bet that you are in the minority. Calcium in milk and milk products is more absorbable and therefore a healthier choice. Cottage cheese, which is a popular low-fat dairy product, contains only 94 mg of calcium per 100 g, which may seem quite low. Many low-fat and non-fat brands of cottage cheese have had their liquid or whey skimmed off, which contains most of the cheese's calcium. Solve this by choosing calcium-enriched brands. You can easily conceal milk and milk products in foods by adding powdered, non-fat milk to casserole dishes.

It is important to distinguish between milk products and dairy products, from the point of view of their calcium content. Because calcium is not soluble in fat, butter and cream (considered dairy products) contain negligible amounts of calcium, while one glass of non-fat milk yields 315 mg of calcium and zero grams of fat! Speaking of fat content, green vegetables would seem to be a better choice if you are watching fat calories, except that some contain binders that inhibit calcium absorption. Dark green leafy vegetables—notably spinach and Swiss chard—inhibit calcium absorption, while kale, parsley and broccoli are better choices.

Recently, attention has been focused on the links between fruit and vegetables and bone health. A report from the World Congress on Osteoporosis 2000 cites studies that suggest a positive association between high consumption of fruit and vegetables and the bone mass of pre-, peri- and postmenopausal women and elderly men. Fruit and vegetables contain high levels of potassium,

magnesium, beta-carotene, fiber and vitamin C, which create an alkaline environment in the body. It is thought that the lack of these nutrients over time increases the breakdown of bone because **calcium salts** are needed to balance the body's acid-base concentration. A well-rounded diet that is rich in fruits, vegetables, milk and milk products will ensure that the ideal amount of calcium is eaten and absorbed into the blood from the intestine.

Calcium Supplements

Some people don't like milk or milk products, or can't eat them because they are **lactose intolerant**. If this is your problem, it is recommended that you take a calcium supplement for your bones, no matter how old you are. The calcium that counts in a supplement is called elemental calcium. Calcium, as a molecule, can't exist alone; it must be attached to another molecule as a salt. Some calcium salts are:

- Calcium carbonate—40 percent calcium
- Calcium citrate—20 percent calcium
- Calcium gluconate—9 percent calcium
- Calcium lactate—13 percent calcium.[3]

Just because you suffer from lactose intolerance doesn't mean that you can't consume calcium-rich foods. Brie, cheddar and cream cheese have low lactose levels, while calcium-fortified orange juice, soy and rice beverages are all lactose-free.

Calcium carbonate contains the most elemental calcium by weight. Some people who have too little stomach acid (achlorhydria) need calcium citrate as a supplement as it is more acid than calcium carbonate and slightly better absorbed. In healthy people, calcium carbonate is just fine as a supplement.

It was found that calcium from the carbonate salt is as fully absorbed from the intestine into the blood as from the citrate salt.[4] Research shows, however, that some calcium carbonate supplements, particularly those made from oyster shells, contained detectable levels of lead, which is harmful to bone.

When buying your calcium supplement, read the label carefully, because it is the elemental calcium that counts when calculating your daily calcium intake. For example, since most calcium carbonate pills are 1250 mg but contain only 500 mg of elemental calcium, you need two tablets daily for 1000 mg or three tablets daily for 1500 mg. Calcium citrate tablets are 1500 mg, containing 300 mg of elemental calcium, so you need three to four tablets daily for 900 to 1200 mg of calcium.

> To test the solubility of your calcium supplement, drop it into a cup of warm water and stir occasionally. A high-quality formulation will dissolve within half an hour.

Pick a calcium supplement that you like, whether it is a tablet, chewable, or flavored. There is now a calcium supplement on the market that is like a caramel or chocolate candy. Share a bottle with a friend or get a sample to try them out. If you like your calcium supplement, you will be much more likely to take it regularly. Keep it in your purse, car, desk or night table drawer.

> Elemental calcium is what counts, so read the label of your supplement carefully. It should also contain vitamin D (see below).

Vitamin D

Vitamin D belongs to a team of hormones and nutrients that work together to produce and maintain bone. It has many functions, all of which help to make calcium and phosphorus available in the blood for the bones to use. Vitamin D helps in the absorption of calcium from the intestine into the blood, making the nutrient available to the bones. Vitamin D increases calcium absorption by 30 to 80 percent and is therefore a vital contributor to bone health. Moreover, vitamin D causes calcium to be retained by the kidneys that would otherwise be lost in the urine, and stimulates osteoclasts to break down bone if blood calcium levels are low.

Vitamin D is as vital to bone development as calcium is. If calcium represents the message, then vitamin D acts as the messenger. Without the messenger, the message is never received and therefore means nothing. In other words, a person can consume large amounts of calcium, but if it can't be absorbed, it will be excreted from the body. Vitamin D helps the body to absorb vital calcium.

Extreme vitamin D deficiency causes rickets in children and osteomalacia in adults. Vitamin D deficiency is common in people who are home- or institution-bound, and in people with dark pigmentation who live in temperate climates during winter months. Vitamin D insufficiency (a mild degree of vitamin D deficiency) is fairly common during the winter months due to lack of sun exposure. Adequate vitamin D intake in winter significantly reduces late-winter bone loss and improves net bone density in postmenopausal women.[5]

Worldwide, the vitamin D deficiency disease rickets still afflicts many children. In rickets, the bones fail to calcify normally and skeletal abnormalities occur. A child with rickets characteristically develops bowed legs because the weak bones bend through support of the body weight.

Vitamin D is obtained by the body in three ways: it can be made by the body with the help of the sun; it can be ingested in food sources; or it can be obtained by taking a supplement.

Vitamin D as a Hormone

Vitamin D is often referred to as a hormone because our bodies produce it in one organ to act on other organs. It is also often referred to as the "sunshine vitamin," because sunlight on our skin helps the body to manufacture its own vitamin D. As little as 15 minutes of daily summer sun exposure can greatly enhance vitamin D production.

Vitamin D goes through numerous conversions before reaching its most potent and active form. It begins in the body as a molecule that is a cousin of cholesterol and is converted to vitamin D_3 (**cholecalciferol**) by ultraviolet rays (UV rays) in the skin. It is then transported to the liver and converted by an enzyme into 25-hydroxycholecalciferol, followed by a trip to the kidney where the final conversion to the active and useful form takes place. This active form is called 1,25-dihydroxycholecalciferol and is 500 to 1000 times stronger than the original precursor. You may be wondering where vitamin D from food sources fits in to all of this. Vitamin D from food enters the body through the intestines as cholecalciferol, which is the same product made after sunlight conversion in the skin.

Lack of Sun and Vitamin D

If only 15 minutes of sun exposure a day can provide you with the necessary vitamin D, then why all the fuss about ensuring adequate consumption? Numerous studies have found that young and old alike are vitamin D deficient, especially during the winter months. It is this deficiency that may cause up to 40 percent of the hip fractures in older people in temperate climates.

Many Americans experience little to no sun exposure during the winter months, and although our bodies can store vitamin D, these resources are quickly depleted after only a couple of days. The little sun that we do receive during the winter is not intense enough to spark the conversion of vitamin D to its active form. Another factor to consider is that, as we age, our skin's ability to react to sun exposure and produce this essential vitamin is less efficient.

A recent study that examined vitamin D levels in individuals whose sunlight exposure is limited focused on the vitamin D status of 69 Moslem women of Arab origin (60 veiled and nine non-veiled) compared to 44 non-veiled age-matched Danish and Danish-Moslem women (all living in Denmark). The veiled Arab women displayed extremely low values of vitamin D compared to their non-veiled counterparts. The veiled women who had higher daily intakes of vitamin D through food consumption had consistently higher levels of the nutrient in their systems, but still had less than the non-veiled women did overall.[6] Although vitamin D intake through the diet is an excellent way to maintain the nutrient's level in the body, one cannot ignore the effect of daily sun exposure on these individuals.

With the increase in cases of skin cancer, our worries about too much sun exposure are warranted. Sun exposure also causes dry skin, wrinkles and sun spots. For sunscreen to be effective, it must be applied 20 to 30 minutes before you go out in the sun. However, while sunscreen protects the skin from harmful UV rays, it also blocks the beneficial rays that convert vitamin D into its active form. If you protect your skin while you're in the sun, be sure to take a vitamin D supplement year-round.

Dietary Sources of Vitamin D

Foods high in vitamin D are hard to find; a few good sources are milk, butter, margarine, egg yolk, cod liver oil, chicken livers and cold-water fish (mackerel, salmon, herring, swordfish and sardines).

Because calcium and vitamin D work together in bone metabolism, it is no surprise that milk is one product chosen to be fortified with vitamin D. The label on a milk carton states that 1 cup of milk provides 25% of the Daily Value which is similar to the U.S. Recommended Daily Allowance. The U.S. Food and Drug Administration permits the fortification with vitamin D of milk and breakfast cereals as well as some other foods.[7] Other milk products (not yogurt) and fortified products such as margarine, some cereals, soy and rice beverages and breakfast drinks are alternative sources of this essential nutrient.

Vitamin D Supplements

The current U.S. Recommended Daily Allowance for vitamin D is 400 IU (international units).

As there are few potent dietary sources of vitamin D, supplementation is essential. Vitamin D as a supplement is available over the counter as multiple-vitamin tablets, or cod or halibut liver oil capsules, which contain 400 IU in each. You can buy vitamin D pills with 250 IU, 500 IU or 1000 IU in each pill. Many calcium supplements also contain 125 IU of vitamin D in each tablet.

A dose of vitamin D greater than 1000 IU daily should not be taken unless prescribed by your doctor. Too much vitamin D can be toxic to bone cells and decrease bone mass. Some people with kidney disease and certain rare bone diseases need vitamin D in very high doses or more potent forms as part of their treatment. A French study showed that vitamin D and calcium supplements reduced the risk of hip fractures in elderly women.[8]

The Bare Bones

- Your skeleton serves as a calcium bank, offering a ready supply of the mineral should your blood calcium level drop. Low calcium intake will deplete your calcium bank.

- Calcium absorption and resorption is tightly regulated by calcitonin, parathyroid hormone and vitamin D.

- Calcium absorption can be impaired by excessive consumption of caffeine, sodium, protein and fiber. Limit your caffeine consumption to two to three cups a day, and avoid using a saltshaker and eating highly processed foods to decrease your sodium intake. Calculate your protein requirements to monitor your protein consumption and finally, watch out for phytic acid content in fiber, which binds to calcium, retarding its absorption.

- Calcium intake recommendations are 1000–1500 mg a day for women and men between the ages of 13 to 50+ years of age.

- The U.S. Recommended Daily Allowance for vitamin D is 400–800 IU for both women and men, depending on age. Remember that vitamin D can be made in the skin with the help of the sun's rays.

- Analyze your diet and lifestyle, then consider a calcium, vitamin D and magnesium supplement from a reputable manufacturer to ensure adequate intake of these bone-building vitamins and minerals.

Three

More Bone Boosters:
Other Nutritional Strategies

Osteoporosis is more than a lack of dietary calcium. Other minerals and nutrients play important roles not only in strengthening bones but in creating an optimal environment for remodelling.

Leslie Beck, RD

Although calcium and Vitamin D are vital to both the prevention and treatment of osteoporosis, other nutrients also play an important role in bone health. This chapter discusses the efficacy of the plant estrogen soy, vitamin K, and the minerals magnesium, potassium, phosphorus and **boron** in the fight against the Silent Thief. None of these nutrients acts alone to increase bone density, but each is a link in a long chain of reactions that facilitate calcium absorption, slow osteoclast activity, and boost the strength of other bone-building nutrients.

Soy: The Plant Estrogen

Soy has received a lot of attention lately because of its high content of plant estrogens. Because the onset of osteoporosis often coincides with the beginning of menopause, the importance of estrogen and its protective qualities is irrefutable.

As mentioned earlier, menopause brings about many changes in the body that can profoundly affect bone density. During this time, estrogen, the body's natural bone protector, is produced at a substantially lower rate. The plant estrogens called **isoflavones**, which are found in soy products, are similar in chemical structure to estrogen and will bind to the estrogen receptors in the body. The chemical structure of isoflavones is nearly identical in structure to the osteoporosis drug ipriflavone, which inhibits osteoclast activity.

A study conducted at the University of Illinois and presented at the 2nd International Symposium of Soy examined the short-term effects of soybean isoflavones on bone in postmenopausal women. Sixty-six postmenopausal women received 40 g of soy protein daily; their bone mineral density was measured after six weeks of this regime. All showed a significant increase in bone mineral content and bone mineral density in the lumbar spine. Although this was a short-term study for evaluating changes in bone, it seems that the **phytoestrogens** in soy products display estrogen-like activity with regard to bone metabolism.

The encouraging thing about soy is that the calcium absorption from it is equivalent to that of milk: approximately 30 to 40 percent of the calcium is absorbed by the body. When choosing soy products as a resource for calcium, take into account the body's **bioavailability**, that is, the ease with which a nutrient is available for absorption by the body. For example, one cup of cooked soybeans contains 175 mg of calcium, but soybeans high in phytate will inhibit the absorption of some of that calcium. Tofu that is precipitated (or clumped together) with magnesium chloride could contain 30 percent less calcium than calcium sulphate-precipitated tofu.[1] It is important to read the product label and understand the calcium content and its bioavailability in the food you consume. Soy products include tofu, fortified soy milk and tempeh (not soy sauce, however).

Bone-Enhancing Minerals and Vitamins

In Chapter 2, you learned about the importance of calcium and vitamin D in maintaining bone health. You learned that calcium is needed to make up the very mineral complex that bone consists of, and that vitamin D aids in the metabolism and absorption of calcium into the bone. Considerable research has recently been done on other bone-enhancing minerals and vitamins that work with calcium and vitamin D to ensure strong and efficient bone metabolism.

Magnesium

Magnesium is necessary for muscle relaxation, transmission of nerve impulses and the breakdown of glucose in the liver so that the glucose can be used for energy. One-half of the body's magnesium is found in the bones, with one-quarter residing in the muscles and the remainder in other soft tissues. The tissues with the highest magnesium concentration are those that are the most metabolically active: the brain, heart, liver and kidney.

Although research indicates that people with diets rich in magnesium have denser bones, few studies have looked at the connection of dietary magnesium intake and bone loss. Magnesium does not directly increase calcium absorption, but the parathyroid hormone, a regulator of bone, is manufactured with the help of magnesium. Osteoporosis sufferers with magnesium deficiency show low levels of vitamin D's most active form. This could be because the enzyme responsible for the conversion from its less active form requires an adequate supply of magnesium.[2] Magnesium deficiency is most often found in individuals who overuse alcohol, suffer from malnutrition or use diuretics.

The U.S. Recommended Daily Allowance (RDA) for magnesium is 325 mg, a level that can easily be reached with the consumption of magnesium-rich foods. Surveys of typical diets have shown that our daily intake is somewhat lower, at 150 to 300 mg without known adverse effects.

Dietary sources rich in magnesium are molasses, nuts, whole grains and fish. Tofu, legumes, seeds, leafy green vegetables and potatoes also contain this nutrient. Because magnesium is mostly found in the husk and germ of whole grains, switching from starchy breads and pastas to whole wheat is the healthier choice. Many calcium supplements include magnesium: check the label for the content.

The following vegetables appear to decrease bone loss: onion, Italian and common parsley, lettuce, tomato, cucumber, arugula, garlic and dill. They were found to be more effective mixed together rather than consumed individually. So here's your chance to have a great, bone-protective salad!

Vitamin K

Vitamin K is a fat-soluble vitamin that is stored in the liver. It is necessary for the formation of osteoid, which, as explained in Chapter 1, is the soft framework of bone before it hardens to form strong new bone. This vitamin is also required for blood clotting and contributes to the production of collagen. A special feature of vitamin K is that it is made by bacteria in the intestinal tract, and as a result, deficiency is quite rare. This nutrient plays an important role in bone metabolism in the making of a bone protein called **osteocalcin**. Vitamin K is directly responsible for converting osteocalcin from its inactive to its active form. Osteocalcin joins with calcium, holding it in place within the bone. Its deficiency leads to impaired mineralization of the bone.

People who have adequate vitamin K in their diet have fewer hip fractures and a higher bone density than people who consume an inadequate amount. Dietary sources of vitamin K are dark green leafy vegetables, soya oil, broccoli, lettuce, cabbage, spinach, green tea, asparagus, oats and whole wheat.

Potassium

Potassium is an **electrolyte**, which is a mineral salt that carries a charge and is always found paired with another electrolyte of opposite charge (e.g., potassium chloride). This electrolyte aids in water balance and distribution, acid-base balance, muscle and nerve cell function and heart and kidney function.

Studies show that elderly men and women whose diet is high in potassium have denser bones in the spine and hips.[3] Moreover, when proper acid balance in the blood is maintained, the body doesn't need to take calcium from the bones into the blood to maintain acid balance.

A diet that is low in potassium and high in sodium causes bone resorption or destruction and loss of calcium in the urine.

Dietary sources of potassium include oranges, potatoes (you must eat the skins), avocados, tomatoes, flounder, bananas, cantaloupe, dried fruits and dairy products. Fruit and vegetables are very high in potassium and vitamin K, so are protective for the bones. Dietary deficiency of this mineral salt is less common than deficiency caused by excessive fluid loss (sweating, diarrhea or urination) or the use of diuretics and laxatives.

Healthy people do not need potassium supplementation.

Phosphorus

Phosphorus is the second most abundant mineral in the body (as you learned in Chapter 2, calcium is the most abundant), and this mineral is part of a major buffer system to balance the body's acid-base levels. It is part of DNA, our genetic material, and is also found in ATP, our body's energy molecule.

Eighty-five percent of the body's phosphorus is found as calcium phosphate, part of the crystal-like substance in bones and teeth that gives them strength and rigidity.[4] Phosphorus plays a dual role in bone health in that extreme levels in the body can positively or negatively affect bone integrity. If phosphorus levels are too high, parathyroid hormone is released, activating the osteoclasts to clear bone, releasing calcium into the bloodstream. If phosphorus levels are too low, bone will also release calcium phosphate to keep blood levels stable.

The U.S. Recommended Daily Allowance (RDA) for phosphorus is 700 mg, which can easily be consumed through diet. Phosphorus deficiencies are next to unknown. Most of us obtain our daily phosphorus in additives found in processed foods like baked products, cereals, processed meats and cheese. Contrary to popular belief, drinking soft drinks does not interfere with calcium absorption. Pop contains a negligible amount of phosphorus (20 to 40 mg) compared to milk (1 cup = 200 mg), demonstrating that you'd have to consume six soft drinks a day to even equal the phosphorus intake associated with drinking milk. Pop only causes concern when it is substituted for calcium-rich beverages in the diet.[5]

Boron

Boron is a trace mineral; in other words, it is found in and needed by the body in small amounts. This mineral has recently attracted much attention in the medical literature because it may be helpful in maintaining healthy bone and joint function. No one knows exactly how boron works in the body; however, evidence since 1980 indicates that it plays a major role in calcium and magnesium metabolism.[6]

Boron is thought to possess mild estrogenic properties by elevating blood estrogen levels after menopause, which is important because, as you have already learned, estrogen is a bone protector. A recent study showed that supplementing the diet of postmenopausal women with 3 mg of boron a day reduced calcium excretion in the urine by 44 percent.[7] Although there are no current RDAs for boron, a safe daily dosage is 9 mg.

Boron can be found in most fruits, including apples, bananas, berries, grapes, pears, cantaloupe and plums.

Boron may play a role in joint health. Boron supplementation has been used in the treatment of osteoarthritis in Germany since the mid-1970s.

Good Overall Nutrition: The Best Strategy

Good nutritional plans not only ensure that you are provided with adequate calories so that you don't lose weight, but also ensure that your intake of dairy products, protein, fruits and vegetables is sufficient to protect muscle mass, enrich your bones, and enhance general health and vigor. Following The *Dietary Guidelines for Americans* and the *Food Guide Pyramid* can help

FOOD GUIDE PYRAMID

KEY
◻ Fat (naturally occurring and added)
▼ Sugars (added)

These symbols show fats
and added sugars in foods.

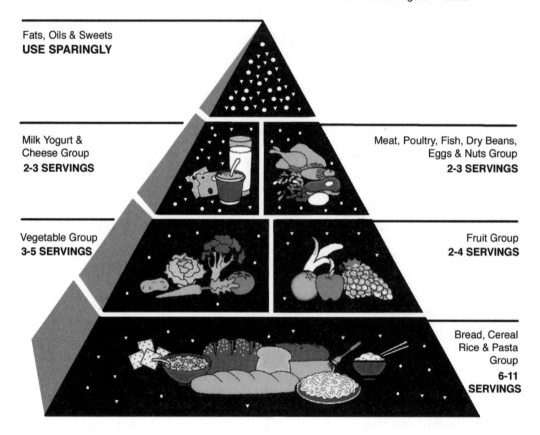

Fats, Oils & Sweets
USE SPARINGLY

Milk Yogurt &
Cheese Group
2-3 SERVINGS

Meat, Poultry, Fish, Dry Beans,
Eggs & Nuts Group
2-3 SERVINGS

Vegetable Group
3-5 SERVINGS

Fruit Group
2-4 SERVINGS

Bread, Cereal
Rice & Pasta
Group
**6-11
SERVINGS**

HOW TO USE THE FOOD GUIDE PYRAMID

What counts as a serving?	How many servings do you need each day?		
	1600 calories*	2200 calories*	2800 calories*
Bread, Cereal, Rice, and Pasta Group • 1 slice of bread • About 1 cup of ready-to-eat cereal • ½ cup of cooked cereal, rice, or pasta	6	9	11
Vegetable Group • 1 cup of raw leafy vegetables • ½ cup of other vegetables—cooked or raw • ¾ cup of vegetable juice	3	4	5
Milk, Yogurt, and Cheese Group **preferably fat free or low fat** • 1 cup of milk *** or yogurt • 1½ ounces of natural cheese (such as Cheddar) • 2 ounces of processed cheese (such as American)	2 or 3**	2 or 3**	2 or 3**

Meat, Poultry, Fish, Dry Beans, Eggs
and Nuts Group—preferably lean or low fat
• 2-3 ounces of cooked lean meat, poultry, or fish
  These count as 1 ounce of meat
  • ½ cup of cooked dry beans or tofu
  • 2½ ounce soyburger
  • 1 egg
  • 2 tablespoons of peanut butter
  • ⅓ cup of nuts
	2, for a total
	of 5 ounces
		2, for a total
		of 6 ounces
			3, for a total
			of 7 ounces

*Recommended number of servings depends on your calorie needs:
• 1600 calories is about right for children ages 2-6 years, many sedentary women, and some older adults.
• 2200 calories is about right for most children over 6, teen girls, active women, and many sedentary men.
• 2800 calories is about right for teen boys and active men.

**Children and teens ages 9 to 18 years and adults over age 50 need 3 servings daily; others need 2 servings daily.

*** This includes lactose-free and lactose-reduced milk products. Soy-based beverages with added calcium are an option for those who prefer a non-dairy source of calcium.

NOTE: Many of the serving sizes given above are smaller than those on the Nutrition Facts Label. For example, 1 serving of cooked cereal, rice, or pasta is 1 cup for the label, but only ½ cup for the Pyramid.

Reprinted from the Dietary Guidelines for Americans, United States Department of Agriculture.

you to achieve a stable, healthy nutritional intake, as well as encouraging you to experiment with varied sources of essential vitamins and minerals. Use it as a rule of thumb when planning your menu, and your overall health is sure to benefit.

The Food Guide Pyramid and the *Dietary Guidelines for Americans,* when used in conjunction with the additional nutritional tips offered in this chapter, will help you to gain an advantage against the Silent Thief. Eat healthily and well!

The Bare Bones

- Soy and soy products contain compounds called isoflavones that mimic the chemical structure and properties of the bone-protecting hormone estrogen.

- Magnesium is the energy-production mineral that is found in bone. Magnesium aids in the activation of the conversion of vitamin D into its most potent and active form. Many calcium supplements include magnesium; check the label.

- Vitamin K plays an important role in bone metabolism by making a bone protein called osteocalcin. This protein joins with calcium and holds it in place within the bone.

- Potassium is an electrolyte that aids in water balance and is thought to help keep proper acid balance in the blood. If balance is maintained, calcium is not pulled from the bones to buffer the imbalance.

- Phosphorus is the second most abundant mineral in the body and is mostly found bound to calcium in bones to give them rigidity. Like calcium, phosphorus levels in the blood must be maintained within specific parameters to ensure bone health.

- Boron is a trace mineral that is thought to aid bone health by helping to metabolize calcium and magnesium. Boron is thought to possess mild estrogenic properties by elevating blood estrogen levels after menopause. This is an important feature, as estrogen is a bone protector.

Four

Drug Strategies to Prevent and Treat Osteoporosis

I started taking Fosamax (alendrondate) in 1997 for my severe osteoporosis. When I had a really bad fall, I cut my lip, and bruised my face, hands, knees and hips. I was quite surprised! I didn't break anything!

—Gertrude Newman, osteoporosis patient

We are at Chapter 4 already! You have learned about your bones and osteo-porosis. You have also learned about the importance of adequate calcium and vitamin D intake for optimal bone health. Next, you will learn about the many drug therapies to prevent and treat osteoporosis.

In the United States, before a drug can be prescribed by your doctor and dispensed by your pharmacist, it must be approved by the United States Food and Drug Administration (FDA). Moreover, the pharmaceutical com-pany that produces the drug must provide scientific evidence that the drug does, in fact, do what is claimed. Some drugs are approved for treatment of osteoporosis only, while others are approved for both treatment and preven-tion. Use this chapter to help you decide which drug therapies to select in outwitting the Silent Thief.

Hormone Replacement Therapy (HRT)

Hormone replacement therapy (HRT), also called **estrogen replacement therapy** (ERT), has been shown to prevent bone loss in postmenopausal women. HRT is approved by the FDA for both the prevention and treatment of osteoporosis. The best time to start learning about HRT is before you reach menopause, which is also a good time to evaluate your overall health. Armed with information about the associated risks, benefits and side effects of HRT, you will be prepared to make a well-informed choice. The decision is between you and your doctor; ultimately, it is *your* choice.

At menopause, women no longer have their menstrual periods because their biological clock stops. The ovaries age and cease making the hormones estrogen, **progesterone** and a small amount of testosterone. They don't quit suddenly; rather, they diminish in function gradually until there is little estrogen left in the body. Heavier women will store estrogen in their fat for several years longer than thinner women.

The definition of menopause is twelve months without a menstrual period. Early menopause occurs when menstrual periods stop or the ovaries are surgically removed (oophorectomy) before age 45. Many women who have had a **hysterectomy** (surgical removal of the womb, or uterus) after age 40 to 45 have had the ovaries removed also.

Symptoms of menopause are of two main types: feeling cold, **hot flashes**, perspiration and insomnia (which affect 75 percent of postmenopausal women and may persist for over five years in 25 percent or may be lifelong in a small minority); and vaginal dryness and thinning.[1] HRT relieves these symptoms of menopause, but it is also considered the therapy of choice for the prevention of osteoporosis because it slows the accelerated bone loss that normally occurs with menopause. There is a 50 percent reduction in fractures if HRT is started early in menopause and continued for six to nine years. Moreover, estrogen prevents further bone loss in older women who are osteopenic or osteoporotic and more than 10 to 15 years postmenopausal. Thus, HRT is useful for both prevention and treatment of osteoporosis. As a treatment for osteoporosis, it is frequently used in combination with another drug, such as a **bisphosphonate** (see page 63).[2]

Benefits, Risks, Contraindications and Side Effects of HRT

Some of the issues around the benefits and risks of hormone replacement therapy are still under debate. As mentioned above, it is important for women considering HRT to examine both risks and benefits before making their decision.

Benefits

There are a number of benefits associated with HRT:

- A decrease in the lifelong probability of fractures
- The alleviation of menopausal symptoms
- Increased life expectancy

It is also thought that HRT decreases the risk of Alzheimer's disease, cataracts and tooth loss, and that it improves the quality of the skin.

HRT was once thought to be totally protective against heart disease in women; currently, however, there is considerable disagreement about this. Thirty studies have shown that there is a 40 to 50 percent decreased risk of heart disease in women on HRT. Hormone replacement therapy decreases **low density lipoprotein** (LDL, or "bad" cholesterol) and increases **high density lipoprotein** (HDL, or "good" cholesterol) in the body. HRT may act as an **antioxidant** (a substance that inhibits another substance from reacting chemically with oxygen, thus preventing tissue damage) and lowers blood pressure slightly. It also appears to strengthen the walls of normal blood vessels.

A PEPI trial[3] found that HRT increases a marker in the blood for inflammation (the marker is a substance in the blood that reflects the presence of tissue injury or destruction). Given that inflammation may play a role in angina and heart attacks, there may be an increased risk of heart disease for women on HRT.

A HERS study[4] indicates that HRT for postmenopausal women did not prevent further heart attacks or death from heart disease if a woman already had heart disease. Dr. Eva Lonn, a cardiologist at the Hamilton Health Sciences Corporation, believes that HRT should not be started in women who have heart disease, but for women already on HRT it is safe to continue HRT. It is best to discuss this with a cardiologist. For women with heart disease, there are other options for treatment of osteoporosis besides HRT, which you will learn about below.[5]

Side Effects

A side effect is a consequence of a drug other than that which is intended; for example, an antibiotic is taken to treat an infection, but it may cause diarrhea or a rash, which are side effects. Side effects of a drug can be mild or extremely serious, to the point of being life threatening. In medicine, really serious side effects can be described as risks.

Consider the following possible side effects of HRT when you are making your decision to take this treatment:

- Bloating
- Headaches
- Breast tenderness
- Vaginal bleeding

Contraindications

There are a number of **contraindications** for hormone replacement therapy that would cause this treatment to be inappropriate. HRT should not be used if you had or currently have: cancer of the breast or uterus (risk of breast cancer increases if a first-degree relative—mother or sister—has or had breast cancer); unexpected or unusual vaginal bleeding; serious liver disease; or blood clots in the legs or lungs.

Risks

The serious risks associated with HRT, which have received considerable coverage, include the following:

Increased lifelong probability of endometrial cancer. In the 1960s, women were put on estrogen alone, which caused the **endometrium** (the lining of the uterus) to thicken and sometimes become cancerous. In 2000, a woman who has her uterus will take as her HRT estrogen (female sex hormone produced by the ovaries and responsible for breast development and sexual maturation of girls) and **progestin** (female sex hormone made in the ovaries and placenta). The main job of progestin is to prepare the lining of the uterus, or womb, to receive and help the development of the fertilized ovum (egg). The progestin also causes the endometrium to shed regularly as a "period" or vaginal bleed. Some schedules for HRT cause the endometrium to shrink away to practically nothing. With the regular shedding or shrinking of the endometrium, the risk of endometrial cancer becomes the same as that for a woman who has never been on HRT. Moreover, when the endometrium shrinks, she won't experience vaginal bleeding. A woman without her uterus does not need progestin.

Increased lifelong probability of breast cancer. Does HRT increase the risk of breast cancer in women who are otherwise not at risk? More than 50 clinical studies that included 350,000 women have looked for a relationship between ERT or HRT and breast cancer. The results of these studies are conflicting and confusing. Most studies have not shown a higher risk of breast cancer in women who have used estrogen at some time in their lives. Some studies suggest that there may be a higher risk of breast cancer in women who use estrogens for ten years or more. The effect on the breast of adding progestin to estrogen is still unclear. Some studies have shown a slightly higher risk in women on estrogen and progestin than with estrogen alone, while others have not. The increased risk remains small for most women and is often outweighed by the benefits of therapy.

By age 60, if women have never taken HRT, 2.4 women of 100 will get breast cancer; if women have taken HRT, 3.3 women of 100 will get breast cancer. By age 85, 10 of 100 women will get breast cancer if they have never taken HRT; if they have taken HRT, 12 to 14 of 100 women will get breast cancer. By age 85, 15 of 100 women will have fractured a hip.

If the reason for taking HRT is to treat menopausal symptoms or prevent osteoporosis, then HRT is the answer. A small number of postmenopausal women should not take HRT, but in the vast majority it is safe.

> Researchers believe that estrogen production decreases at menopause; thus there is a change in brain chemistry that affects the temperature control center in the hypothalamus (the body's thermostat).

Taking HRT

If after considering all sides of the HRT issue you decide to take hormone replacement therapy, you will need:

- An annual mammogram
- An annual breast examination by your doctor
- A monthly breast self-examination (BSE)
- An annual pelvic examination with a Pap smear—a sample of the cells of the cervix (the lower part of the uterus or womb) to detect cancer

Now you are ready for HRT. As mentioned above, HRT consists of an estrogen and a progestin. If you have had a hysterectomy, you only need estrogen. Estrogen preparations can be taken orally, vaginally, or by injection, or can be applied to the skin as a gel or patch. Progestin is taken by mouth or as a patch on the skin. As you can see, there are a number of options open to you. HRT can be tailored to you and your needs, to ensure the fewest side effects and lowest risks. Work with your doctor to come up with the combination that you are most comfortable with.

If you have to stop HRT for any reason, go off it gradually; otherwise, you may experience menopausal symptoms. Replace the HRT with another bone-protective drug, as stopping HRT leads to rapid loss of bone mineral density.

Selective Estrogen Receptor Modulators (SERMs)

A **selective estrogen receptor modulator (SERM)**, raloxifene (Evista) is approved for the prevention and treatment of osteoporosis. Used for many years to treat breast cancer, the drug **tamoxifen** was the first SERM to be developed. It is important to note that SERMs are not estrogens. They are totally different compounds with different chemical structures. They sometimes act like estrogen, while at other times they block the effects of estrogen. This is why they are said to be "selective." Raloxifene affects the bone and heart in a similar way to estrogen, while it does not have the undesirable estrogen effects on the uterus and breasts. In a study, raloxifene was shown to improve bone mineral density by 2.4 percent and reduce the number of vertebral fractures by 35 percent when taken for two years.

Raloxifene is taken daily as a 60 mg pill. Like hormone therapy, raloxifene is only effective on your bones while you are taking it. Side effects include leg cramps, hot flashes and blood clots, particularly in women with a previous history or risk factors for blood clots.

Women with a history of breast cancer or who are still menstruating should not take raloxifene. It has a positive effect on several risk factors for heart disease by reducing LDL (the bad cholesterol) and total cholesterol.[6]

Calcitonin

In humans, calcitonin is made by the thyroid gland and acts by inhibiting bone removal by the osteoclasts. Calcitonin is approved as a treatment for osteoporosis by injection or nasal spray.

Calcitonin (Miacalcin NS) is given as one 200 IU spray administered inside the nose to alternating nostrils daily. It can be taken at any time of day with few side effects except for the rare side effect of a runny nose. A study indicates that nasal spray calcitonin decreases the number of vertebral fractures by 36 percent and increases the bone mineral density of the vertebrae by 2.4 percent when given for two years. It is also available as an injection (50-100 IU) daily with the possible side effects of flushing, nausea and skin rash.

Both nasal spray and injectable calcitonin have a role in pain management after an acute vertebral fracture. Nasal spray calcitonin has been shown to reduce the time spent in bed and the number of analgesics (pain relievers) taken after an acute vertebral fracture.[7]

Bisphosphonates

Bisphosphonates were first made in 1865 to be used as an antiscaling agent. A major advance has been the development and introduction of bisphosphonates for use in osteoporosis therapy. In 2000, they are the treatment of choice for bone diseases that involve removal of too much bone by the osteoclasts. Bisphosphonates act by binding to the mineral surface in bone and interfering with the bone-chewing action of the osteoclasts, thus decreasing bone resorption (bone removal or destruction) and bone loss.

In the United States two bisphosphonates have been approved by the FDA as effective therapies for the prevention and treatment of osteoporosis: alendronate and risedronate. These drugs are considered the number-one choice as they act specifically on bone cells and show the best evidence that they improve bone mineral density and decrease the number of fractures. Essentially all studies on bisphosphonates were done on postmenopausal women, but studies in men with osteoporosis are in progress.

Alendronate and Risedronate

Alendronate (Fosamax) and risedronate (Actonel) are intensively researched drugs which contain a nitrogen molecule that makes the drugs very strong. They act by interfering with enzymes that are involved in making proteins inside the osteoclasts. These proteins play a key role in signaling the osteoclast to ruffle its membrane and produce bone-destroying acid that removes bone. A point of great interest is that these enzymes are on the same pathway that makes cholesterol in the liver, but these drugs are very specific to bone.

Studies have shown that alendronate and risedronate build healthy bone by increasing bone mineral density by 7 to 9 percent and reducing the number of vertebral and non-vertebral fractures by 35 to 50 percent over two years.

Alendronate (Fosamax) is approved for prevention as a 5 mg tablet daily or 35 mg once a week. For treatment of osteoporosis alendronate (Fosamax) is approved for treatment as a 10 mg tablet daily or 70 mg once a week. Risedronate (Actonel) is approved for prevention and treatment as a 5 mg tablet daily.

Bisphosphonates are poorly absorbed from the intestine. Food and medications reduce their absorption, as does stomach acidity. Bisphosphonates should be taken with tap water only, on an empty stomach; do not eat, drink or take other medications for at least 30 minutes or according to the specific directions for the drug that you are taking. Once absorbed from the intestine, bisphosphonates are cleared from the blood in minutes. Half of the drug stays in the skeleton and half is excreted in the urine. Bisphosphonates stay in the skeleton for as long as ten years or more.

Side effects of oral bisphosphonates include nausea, abdominal pain and diarrhea. A very few people develop a skin rash. Some people report an irritated or ulcerated esophagus, mainly from alendronate, but this is rare if the drug is taken properly.[8]

A lot of research is being done into new and better treatments for osteoporosis, such as parathyroid hormone and new bisphosphonates. Stay tuned!

Bone mineral density should be monitored every two years in people who are being treated for osteoporosis, as about 10 to 20 percent don't respond to drug therapy as expected. If you do not respond to drug therapy, then you could be treated for another two years and be retested, or another agent could be added to your drug regime, such as hormone replacement therapy, a SERM or calcitonin.

The ultimate purpose of the prevention and treatment of osteoporosis is to reduce lifetime disease and death from fractures, which are the consequences of osteoporosis. This may sound gloomy, but it really is the bottom line.

Hip fracture is the most serious consequence of a fall. Despite successful surgical results, approximately 60 percent of those with a hip fracture become less mobile.

A Plan for You

Now that you are armed with useful information to help you outwit the Silent Thief, consider the following plan of action to further prevent and treat osteoporosis and to stop fractures.

- Modify your risk factors with an adequate daily intake of calcium and vitamin D, and by exercising, stopping smoking and reducing alcohol intake.

- If you are at risk for osteoporosis or a fracture or have had a fracture after age 40, get a bone mineral density test.

- If you are at low risk of fracture or have had a bone mineral density test that shows you to be osteopenic but not osteoporotic, consider

HRT, a SERM or nasal calcitonin to prevent further bone loss. Have a repeat bone mineral density test in three to five years to be sure that your bones are remaining strong and healthy.

- If your bone mineral density shows you to have osteoporosis or osteopenia and you have had a fracture, drug therapy should be started. The best choice is a bisphosphonate, especially a potent, nitrogen-containing one such as alendronate or risedronate.

- One to two years after starting drug therapy for osteoporosis, have a repeat bone mineral density test. If your BMD has remained the same or improved, then your treatment is doing the job that you and your doctor want it to do. If your BMD has decreased by 3 percent or more, then you have not responded as expected to therapy, and another drug can be added to your current regime. If your osteoporosis is being managed by your family doctor, this might be a good time to see a specialist in osteoporosis to assist with the additions or changes to your therapy.

DRUG STRATEGIES TO PREVENT AND TREAT OSTEOPOROSIS

Many drug therapies are now available for the prevention and treatment of osteoporosis. Here are some of your options:

For Prevention

- hormone replacement therapy (HRT)
- selective estrogen receptor modulators (SERMs): raloxifene
- calcitonin (nasal spray, injectable)
- bisphosphonates: alendronate; risedronate

For Treatment

- bisphosphonates: alendronate; risedronate
- hormone replacement therapy (HRT)
- selective estrogen receptor modulators (SERMs): raloxifene
- calcitonin (nasal spray, injectable)

The Bare Bones

- The definition of menopause is 12 months without a menstrual period. The use of hormone replacement therapy (HRT) is associated with a decrease in the number of vertebral fractures. Estrogen prevents further bone loss in older women who are osteopenic or osteoporotic or more than 10 to 15 years postmenopausal.

- Common risks associated with taking HRT include an increased life-long probability of endometrial cancer and an increased lifelong probability of breast cancer.

- If you decide to take HRT, you should have, initially and annually, a mammogram, a breast examination by your doctor and a pelvic examination with a Pap smear. You should learn to do a breast self-examination (BSE) and perform it monthly.

- The hormone calcitonin is made by the thyroid gland and acts to inhibit bone removal by the osteoclasts. This treatment is now available in nasal spray form.

- Bisphosphonates have become the treatment of choice for bone diseases that involve too much bone removal by the osteoclasts. In the United States, two bisphosphonates have been approved for prevention and treatment of osteoporosis: alendronate (Fosamax) and risedronate (Actonel).

Outwitting the Silent Thief with Exercise

Five

Exercise: The Magic Cure?

My main motivation behind starting an exercise program was to improve bone health. If I had known that exercise could decrease my stress levels, reduce my risk of heart disease and make me feel better, I would have started years ago.

—Linda Coleman, personal training client

Now that you know how to fortify your body nutritionally to outwit the Silent Thief, you are ready to learn how you can use exercise to prevent osteoporosis, or how exercise can make it easier to live with the disease if you already have it.

As we age, our activity levels decline along with our physical strength and overall **fitness**. The modern world has contributed to a trend among adults that has them adopting an increasingly sedentary lifestyle. Children, too, have become less active, as physical education programs at school are curtailed due to government budgetary cuts and as the temptations of modern technology—computers and the Internet, for example—have them doing more sitting and less running, jumping and learning new sports.

Some call exercise "the magic cure," but there is nothing magic about it. It's all science, but don't let that scare you. Once you learn which activities exercise which systems and why, you'll be on your way to understanding how you can exercise to improve bone health and guard yourself against osteoporosis.

Other Benefits of Exercise

- Helps prevent high blood pressure (hypertension), cardiovascular disease and high cholesterol
- Increases muscle tone
- Lowers body fat, which means a leaner body
- Strengthens the immune system
- Relieves stress, thus improving overall mental health
- Increases self confidence as challenging exercises become easier to perform
- Improves quality of life as everyday tasks become easier to complete

Key Components of Fitness

Exercise improves overall fitness. The term "fitness" refers to the health of the many components in our bodies. These components include the **cardiores-**

piratory system, muscular strength, muscular endurance and flexibility. Whether we work these systems together or individually, each ultimately affects the others. Running, for example, challenges the heart and lungs, uses muscular strength to propel the body forward and uses muscular endurance to keep it going. Flexibility plays a part in preventing injuries associated with any activity. Being fit means that all of these components are healthy, allowing us to participate in everyday activities with energy and vitality.

Cardiorespiratory System

The cardiorespiratory system is the body's transport network. It consists of the heart, lungs, arteries, capillaries and veins. The lungs inhale oxygen, the heart pumps oxygen-containing blood through the arteries to the cells in the body and the veins carry the oxygen-depleted blood back to the heart. The cardiorespiratory system improves with exercise when you participate in **aerobic activities**. "Aerobic" simply means "oxygen-using," and aerobic activities increase the demand for oxygen delivery to the working muscles.

Aerobic activities include walking, running, swimming, cycling and dancing. These activities engage the whole body, especially the large muscle groups, in oxygen-demanding movements that raise the heart rate. My osteoporotic clients engage in aerobic activities that benefit the skeletal system while improving their cardiovascular fitness. Aerobic conditioning will make your whole body a more efficient machine.

Muscular Strength

Muscular strength refers to a muscle's ability to exert force against resistance during a muscular contraction. Muscular strength improves when you place a demand or overload on the muscles in a way that you're not accustomed to. If the overload is applied safely and progressively, the muscular system will adapt and as a result you will become stronger.

Muscular strength is area-specific, which means that it can vary at different sites on the body. Resistance training or lifting weights is the best way to increase muscular strength at all the different sites. Resistance training can be done using machines, dumbbells, elastic **exercise bands** or your own body weight. Everyday activities—like getting out of a chair, lifting a child and pushing open a door—require muscular strength. Resistance training will increase lean muscle mass, strengthen bones and make everyday activities easier to complete.

Muscular Endurance

Muscular endurance is the body's ability to keep doing an activity while resisting muscular fatigue. When you can keep up repeated muscular contractions of the same activity and **intensity** for longer periods of time, your muscular endurance has improved. Lifting heavy grocery bags requires muscular strength, but carrying those bags over a distance requires muscular endurance. Improved muscular endurance allows you to participate for a longer time in demanding activities. I challenge my clients' muscular endurance with specific resistance-training drills that keep their muscles contracting to the point of fatigue.

Flexibility

Flexibility is defined as the range of motion available around a joint. A flexible joint is able to move freely in every direction. Because ligaments and tendons have little or no elasticity, flexibility often depends on the lengthening of muscle. When you stretch, you take the joint slightly beyond the normal range of motion and hold it at that position. This will lengthen the muscles and increase the range of motion, allowing the joint to move more freely. Maintaining flexibility is important for preventing injuries and free movement during everyday activities.

Exercise and the Silent Thief

Whether you are 70 years old and diagnosed with osteoporosis, or 30 years old and have been exposed to the disease through your mother or grandmother, exercise that you participate in today affects osteoporosis. The effectiveness of exercise is not restricted to a particular age group. For older individuals living with osteoporosis, an appropriate exercise program can stop bone loss due to aging. For young people, a well-rounded resistance and weight-bearing workout can contribute to forming and maintaining peak bone mass in earlier years, giving you a head start in preventing osteoporosis.

Can Exercise Prevent Osteoporosis?

Exercise can prevent many things, and osteoporosis is one of them. In preventing the disease, exercise contributes to reaching peak bone mass and increasing strength, and thereby preventing fractures. Obtaining optimal peak bone mass at a young age is vital in preventing osteoporosis. Exercise puts positive stress on the bones while strengthening the muscles that support them. A stronger body means stronger bones, thus preventing fractures, especially in the hip, spine and wrist. Postmenopausal women showed significant increases in hip and spinal bone mineral density after they participated in a biweekly, year-long, high-intensity resistance-training program.[1] Exercise also plays an important role in warding off the debilitating effects of osteoporosis. For an osteoporotic person, a fall can result in a fracture that might not heal, further limiting mobility. Exercise can prevent falls by increasing muscular strength, balance, stability and flexibility. It also increases the individual's confidence with daily movements, which diminishes the fear of falling.

Can Exercise Treat Osteoporosis?

Exercise has been proven to slow bone loss and help maintain bone mass. In fact, some research shows that exercise can even increase bone mass. Many studies show higher bone mass in athletes compared to the bone mass of inactive people of the same age. Female professional tennis players were found to have greater overall bone mass than age-matched casual tennis players.[2] These studies show a positive correlation between active lifestyle and bone density, but more research needs to be focused on the effects of exercise on the bones of our aging population. Several studies show that exercise slows bone loss, and in some instances exercise increased bone mass in older women who began exercise programs in their sixties.[3] One fact is sure: a marked decline in physical activity, which often accompanies the aging process, increases the rate of bone loss.

For someone with osteoporosis, exercise can strengthen bones, increase mobility, relieve symptoms, treat back pain and increase quality of life. Individuals who participate in exercise programs experience most of these physiological benefits. They also see visible changes in their muscle tone and feel the challenge of working the muscles. Well, it doesn't end at the muscles. In fact, working the muscle is only the first step in a chain of reactions that ends with stronger bones!

Changing Bones

As discussed in Chapter 1, bones are living tissues. They constantly renew themselves through the remodeling process, with the bone being broken down by osteoclasts and built up by osteoblasts. Exercise is one of the known initiators of bone remodelling.

The continual renewal of bone has a number of physiologically important functions. First, bone will adjust its strength in proportion to the degree of stress placed upon it. Consequently, bones thicken when subjected to heavy loads. Second, even the shape of the bone can change, rearranging the build-up of bone to accommodate particular load patterns. For example, an individual with an injured left knee will change walking and stepping patterns to accommodate the injury, causing the right leg to assume an additional load; osteoblasts will respond by depositing bone in the right leg to accommodate the greater weight. Third, because new bone is needed to replace the old, the normal toughness of bone is maintained.[4]

Inactivity

We now know that bone mineral is deposited in proportion to the load or stress that the bone must carry. If this is the case, then what happens with inactivity when the bones are not challenged? It makes sense that when bone is not continually physically stressed, the remodeling process slows. For instance, bone density in athletes is far greater than in non-athletes, and a broken leg in a cast for weeks results in a thin, decalcified leg bone upon removal of the cast. Although the individual effects of exercise on increasing bone density vary from person to person, there is one fact about exercise and bone density that is unarguable: noticeable decline in physical activity will result in a significant decline in bone density. A decline in physical activity decreases the overall muscle mass of the body and the physical strength that goes along with it. The combination of aging and a sedentary lifestyle results in a functional loss of muscle and, therefore, weaker bones.

Walking is a great exercise for your heart, but no study has ever shown that a middle-aged or older woman can increase her bone density by taking up walking. Short-term effects of walking on bones are minor.

Skeletal Fitness

Exercises specific to fighting osteoporosis can be divided into three categories: resistance training; weight-bearing or impact exercises; and **balance-stability** training. The exercises contained in this book provide programs for all three categories. Below are descriptions of the three categories and a discussion of how participation in the activity can help to maintain your bone mineral density.

Resistance Training

Resistance training or strength training places the needed stresses on specific sites of the body. When you strength-train, you challenge one muscle group at a time by moving a weight against gravity. When a particular muscle is stressed, it pulls on the tendon that attaches it to the bone, sending the bone a message that it needs to respond. The response will be increased activity in the osteoblasts, which are responsible for laying down new bone. Osteoporosis is defined by low bone density. As mentioned earlier, low bone mineral density is site-specific and the activity of resistance training is area-specific. Do you see the connection? For example, if you have osteoporosis, you may have low bone mineral density in a particular area, in the wrist, for example; because weight training is area-specific, you can train the muscles around the wrist and effectively strengthen the very bones that attach to those muscles.

A study showed a bone mineral density difference of 14 percent in the playing arms of 13 competitive tennis players compared to their unused arms. This difference did not change over a four-year period, even though the athletes' competitive careers and strenuous training schedules ended two to three years before the follow-up measurements.[5] This brings up an important point about prevention through exercise. Look at your bones in the way that you look at an IRA. The more you invest and the earlier you start, the bigger your plan will be at the time of retirement. Regular exercise can build bone density in younger years, maximizing peak bone mass and contributing to the prevention of osteoporosis and fractures in later years. Consider the yearly IRA tax break you get from your investments as equal to the shorter-term benefits of exercise, such as weight loss, toned muscles and increased energy!

> Because weight training is about working muscle groups individually, divide your workout into a few shorter sessions throughout the day, making it more time-convenient.

A well-rounded strength-training program is important for an overall balanced body, but the good news is that specific exercises can target specific areas that are prone to low bone density and fractures.

Weight-Bearing Exercises

Weight-bearing exercise simply means supporting your own body weight while doing an activity. Weight-bearing or impact exercises exert pressure on the bones through body-weight support, stressing the skeleton. Most weight-bearing exercises are done standing up and include running, dancing, skipping, jumping and stair climbing. The intensity of the impact of a particular activity will directly affect the stress placed on the bones. For example, running places a higher level of stress on the skeleton than walking because of the greater intensity on the leg, spine and hips when the foot strikes the ground.

Researchers in Australia looked at the relationship between weight-bearing activities and bone mineral density. This study examined three contrasting groups of mature female athletes (42 to 50 years old) with greater than 20 years of training in their particular sport. The three sports were divided into:

(1) high-impact—basketball, netball; (2) medium-impact—running, field hockey; and (3) non-impact—swimming. The bone mineral densities of the women in these groups were compared to each other and to a non-exercising control group of the same age. The results showed: a significantly higher whole body bone mineral density in the high-impact group; a higher level of overall bone mineral density in the medium-impact group compared to the non-impact and non-exercising group; and a higher arm bone mineral density in all three groups compared to the non-exercising group.[6] This study shows the strong correlation between bone density and the intensity of the impact activity.

> Weight training can increase your body's efficiency in burning fat. Your body burns its fat in the muscles. If you picture your muscles as your fuel-burning furnace, it makes sense that the bigger the furnace (the more muscles you have), the more fuel you'll burn!

You might be surprised that swimming is considered a non-impact activity. Swimming is a fabulous way to aerobically work your heart, therapeutically train injuries and increase your range of motion. Water creates a weightless medium, however, which is unfavorable for impacting the bones.[7] If swimming is your activity of choice, please continue but be sure to add weight-bearing activities to your exercise regime.

Balance-Stability Training

"Balance" is defined as equilibrium or steadiness; poise equal to any opposing force. "Stability" is steadiness having permanence, or tending to return to the original position. The common denominator in both of these definitions is the word "steadiness." Steadiness encompasses both the ability to resist movement and the ability to regain a position when moved. We take balance-stability for granted because as we perform our everyday activities, we are unaware of all the bodily controls at play. These controls are very complex, and as we age, their deterioration contributes to instability and lack of confidence in our movements.

A study looked at 110 elderly men and women who were given balance training drills to work through for three months.[8] The study showed that, at the end of three months, the participants had a level of body control and posture stability similar to that of people three to ten years younger. Balance training for the elderly awakens reflexes and teaches body awareness on a subconscious level. This leads to increased confidence in movements and overall quality of movement. On a neurological level, balance training sensitizes special receptor cells called proprioceptors found in the skin, muscles, joints and tendons.[9] These cells process information about the body's orientation in space. To keep it simple, here are the steps involved in maintaining balance:

- Receptors on the skin and in the muscles and joints send a message to the brain about body position; this system is called proprioception—your sense of where you are in space
- Eyes visually interpret information from the environment and send it to the brain
- Equilibrium centers in the brain send messages through the nervous system to the muscles
- Muscles respond by contracting or lengthening to maintain stability and balance; this is done by your body's motor response system

These systems all act to keep you moving, keep you standing and help you to react to sudden changes in body position. Have you ever stumbled on a curb because you have misjudged its height? Your eyes saw the curb as lower than it was and sent a message to the leg muscles to lift the foot, but not high enough. Your foot hits the curb and you start to fall forward. Your proprioceptor cells sense the sudden change in body position and send a message to the brain. Your eyes see the ground coming toward you and they send the information to the brain. The brain tells the muscles to react and regain balance, preventing a fall. The second half of that process is called the **reflex**. The term "quick reflex" can be used to describe your body's ability to react quickly to a sudden external force or situation.

Practicing Your Balance

Balance is a skill that needs to be practiced regularly. Improving balance-stability can reduce the risk of falls and resulting fractures. For an individual with osteoporosis, steadiness is what really matters because it is important for the prevention of falls. A fall that causes a bone fracture can be devastating for a person with osteoporosis as it leads to further inactivity, which can result in other chronic diseases and weaker bones. One way that exercise prevents falls is by increasing an individual's muscular strength. Stronger muscles will support the body, protect the bones and react quickly to sudden changes in body position.[10]

Stand sideways, close to the countertop in your kitchen, with one hand on top. Place your feet in line, one in front of the other, with the heel of the front foot up against the toes of the back one. Close your eyes, lift the hand a few inches above the counter and try to maintain the position for 10 seconds. If you are successful, your balance is pretty good. But remember, there is always room for improvement!

What many people don't know is that a sense of steadiness can be increased through specific balance-training exercises. When we were younger, we challenged and improved our balance by engaging in many activities. A simple game of "pin the tail on the donkey" or walking across a stream on a log tested and increased our sense of balance. If we go back even further, when we first learned to stand on our own without falling, the body laid down the necessary visual, neural and muscular pathways for balance through the repetition of the movements. The point I'm trying to make is that practice makes perfect!

As we age, many factors influence our sense of steadiness. As we become less active, we lose the muscle mass needed to support our skeleton. As our vision deteriorates, we lose one of the most important information tools for balance. This often affects our confidence in performing activities, which only adds to our state of inactivity. Balance exercises are those that simply mimic unstable conditions in a safe environment. The more you train your body to handle imbalance, the better equipped you'll be to avoid a fall.

Exercise Frequency and Intensity

Once you have learned the specific exercises that combat osteoporosis, it is important to know when to do them, how often and at what level. To reap the positive benefits of exercise, you must challenge the body beyond normal everyday activity. Applying the program in a safe, regular and intense fashion is the best way to get fit while strengthening your bones.

Frequency

When discussing exercise, frequency simply means how often. Earlier we learned that physical inactivity has been implicated in bone loss, which suggests that the frequency with which you exercise is important. A recovery period is essential to avoid overtraining and injuries while you are progressively improving your muscular strength. A minimum of 24 hours has been suggested as an adequate recovery period between most exercises. A 48-hour period of rest should be given to any of the resistance-training exercises. These exercises overload the muscle fibers in a building process that needs time to heal. An optimal frequency for resistance training is two to three times a week, challenging all muscle groups.

The frequency with which you perform an exercise in combination with others in your program is also important. The body's muscles overlap and intertwine, which makes the isolation of just one muscle difficult. For example, the chest muscles (pectorals) insert at the front of the shoulder where the anterior deltoid muscle is located. If you performed a push-up exercise for the pectoral muscles, which requires the anterior deltoid to act also, followed by a forward shoulder raise for the anterior deltoid, you have not given the adequate recovery period to the frontal shoulder muscle. Combining exercises in an order that challenges unrelated muscle groups, back to back, will ensure adequate recovery periods and save time; while one muscle recovers, you can be exercising another. An organized system is provided in Chapter 7 to ensure that your program design and order of exercises follows all the recovery rules.

Intensity

Intensity refers to the amount of stress that an activity places on a muscle. How hard you work your muscles is just as important as the frequency with which you do the exercise. For individuals with osteoporosis, exercise intensity must exceed normal bone stress and be continuous in order for bone to grow. Exceeding normal bone stress means that the exercise must challenge the body beyond everyday activities. Unlike frequency, intensity levels are subjective; they are based on the person performing the activity. For a sedentary person, a simple walk around the block can be intense, but for a frequent jogger, the same walk might be used for the warm-up.

The easiest way to measure intensity is to be aware of the way you feel when you exercise. When you perform resistance-training exercises, it is important for you to know what muscle group you're working, what those muscles should feel like during the movement and when to increase the intensity to a new level.

Do you feel overwhelmed by all this information? Don't worry, the next chapter will give you a step-by-step approach to designing an exercise program that incorporates all the aspects of fitness with optimal frequency and intensity.

Effects of Overtraining

Can too much exercise be harmful to your bones? Women who participate in excessive and extreme exercise programs run the risk of losing bone density. Activities such as long-distance running can cause **amenorrhea**, the cessation of menstruation due to loss of body fat. This condition plays an important role in bone density because of the loss of bone-protecting estrogen. In 1990, a four-year study on 97 amenorrheaic female athletes, ages 18 to 38, compared their bone density to a control group of the same age. The athletes had a significantly lower spinal bone density than the control group. Their bone density increased 6 percent in 14 months when activity levels decreased and weight was gained.[11] The 6-percent increase should not be considered an indication of future bone density levels in those individuals because the damage may already have been done. Remember that peak bone density is reached between the ages 18 to 25, and if that is compromised you are already playing catch-up.[12]

As with most things, moderation is the key. A balanced exercise program that challenges all the aspects of fitness will reward you safely.

The Bare Bones

- The four components of fitness are: cardiorespiratory health, muscular strength, muscular endurance and flexibility.

- Bones are living tissues that change in response to stresses placed upon them or decreased activity levels.

- Exercise can prevent osteoporosis by contributing to peak bone mass and muscular strength. High peak bone mass builds up your bank of calcium in preparation for withdrawals in later years. Increased muscular strength prevents fractures by protecting the bones and increasing balance to prevent falls.

- Physical inactivity increases the rate of bone loss. A marked decline in physical activity is often a product of the aging process. Inactivity results in weaker muscles that no longer put the needed demands on the skeleton while decreasing balance and stability that contribute to falls leading to fractures.

- The three types of exercise that profoundly affect the skeleton are resistance training, weight-bearing (or impact) exercises and balance-stability training. Resistance training affects the muscles that support the bones; impact training affects the skeleton; balance training reduces risk of falls leading to fractures.

- Frequency and intensity play an important role in maintaining the positive effects of exercise on osteoporosis. Exercise on a frequent basis (two to four times a week) and challenge your body beyond the intensity of everyday activities to experience the positive, bone-strengthening effects of exercise.

Six

Getting With the Program

One of the things I tell people I work with is that it's not just enough to keep doing the same program. Your body adapts to the stresses you place upon it when working out. You have to keep introducing new things to your program. Either increase the weight or add a few repetitions, and keep the body guessing—this way you won't get bored.

—Phil Delaire, personal trainer

Whether you already exercise or not, incorporating a new program into your daily routine requires careful consideration. Among other things, it is important to think about the commitment you are about to make and the time you're going to spend strengthening your bones. This chapter will familiarize you with exercise terminology, motivate you to prioritize your workouts and give you the tools to advance to new levels of fitness.

Take time to perform your stretches properly. Stay warm by putting on a sweater or sweatshirt, maybe dim the lights, and get rid of any distractions. The sense of relaxation you feel when you are done will be your reward.

Progression

Progression is defined as advancement, headway, development, growth and improvement. Proper progression is the most fundamental concept for success in your exercise program. In Chapter 5, you learned that exercise intensity must exceed normal bone stress and must be continuous in order for bone to grow. Exercise progression challenges the body's abilities gradually, allowing the muscles, in particular, to adapt safely to new intensities. For example, participation in a new activity often causes muscle soreness during the 24 hours that follow. The next time you do the activity (within a week), the soreness is not quite as bad. This is your body adapting to the movements involved. Eventually the activity doesn't challenge the muscles as much anymore, there is no soreness, and the activity seems to take less effort to complete. It is at this point that your body fails to experience all the benefits of exercise. You need to progress to the next level to continue feeling the benefits.

Although muscle soreness can often be attributed to intense physical training, it can also be a result of dehydration. An average person loses 48 ounces of water a day through the pores, urine and breath. If you are exercising on a regular basis, you need to replenish this loss by drinking more than 48 ounces of water a day. Get drinking!

Applying progression to your program will:

- Constantly challenge the body in different ways
- Allow muscles to get stronger as they adapt to new loads
- Eliminate boredom as you learn new exercises and skills
- Decrease the occurrence of injury that is often due to overtraining (too much too soon) and establish goals to work towards

DEFINING TERMS

Resistance   The amount of weight or load placed upon a specific muscle group. Resistance devices can come in the form of a dumbbell, elastic exercise band or your own body weight moving against gravity.

Rep (Repetition)   The term used to describe one complete move from start position to finish and back to start again. One move takes the muscle through contraction (shortening) and relaxation (lengthening). You will complete 8–15 reps.

Sets   A predetermined number of reps make up one set. In the case of the exercises in this book, 8–15 reps will make up one set. You will being doing two sets of each exercise during one workout.

Establishing baseline   Whenever you begin a new exercise, it is important to set a baseline level. This process involves measuring your effort. The baseline level should challenge the muscle you want to work. It should be challenging to complete the set and the muscle should feel fatigued when you are finished working it. Setting a baseline gives you a point of reference from which to progress.

How Do I Know When to Progress?

Understanding which muscle group you're working, knowing where to feel it and how to gauge your effort are all skills you will learn in this section of the book. For example, let's take the bicep curl exercise (see page 104). This exercise works the bicep muscle, which is situated between the shoulder and elbow on the front side of the arm. When performing the bicep curl, you should feel it in the belly of the muscle (the middle of a muscle is often referred to as the "belly"), the center point between the shoulder and elbow. So how should the exercise feel? This involves measuring effort and is a little more difficult to explain because it is so subjective. To measure your effort, use a scale of 1 to 5; 1 represents very little effort, and 5 represents a challenge to complete the task. When a particular exercise, over time, becomes an **effort level** of 2, it is time to progress to the next level. This next level should challenge the muscle at an effort of 4–5. The time between progressions will vary from person to person, but a safe amount of time would be every three to four weeks if you're doing the program two to three times a week. Remember that progressing too quickly may result in injuries. Listen to your body—it's not a race!

When exercising, be sure to wear comfortable, breathable and nonrestrictive clothing. Cotton blends are comfortable and materials like lycra are quick-drying.

How Do I Progress?

If you flip to Chapter 7, you will see that I have provided two or three different exercises for each muscle group. I have labeled each exercise as beginner, intermediate or advanced. It seems obvious that you will want to progress from beginner through to advanced, but progression will also be applied within each category.

For the purpose of this program, you will progress three ways: increasing reps, increasing load (resistance) and changing the exercise. First, increasing reps simply means that you need to complete more reps within each set of the exercise. This will increase your muscular endurance as you resist fatigue while performing more reps. Second, increasing the load means that you may complete the same number of reps but with a heavier weight. The increased load will stress the muscle and supporting bones in a fashion that will demand adaptation. Third, changing the exercise will strengthen the same muscle while challenging it in a different way.

Working your muscles in different planes and positions will improve balance and coordination. Your muscles have a memory like a computer circuit that sends messages through nerves between the brain and muscles. It is this memory that enables you to hop on a bike and ride it after many years of not riding. When you perform the same movement repeatedly over a period of time, your muscles don't have to work as hard to complete a movement they are comfortable doing. This is the reason that it is important to change the exercises. Applying all three progressive techniques will keep your program new and exciting. Consult the following flow chart for the rules of progression.

Progression Flow Chart

Always start with the beginner exercise. Establish a baseline at a resistance where you can complete 8–10 reps at an effort level of 4–5.

↓

When this becomes an effort level of 1–2, increase the number of reps to 12–15 doing the same exercise.

↓

When this becomes an effort level of 1–2, increase the resistance to an effort level of 4–5 at 8–10 reps.

↓

When this becomes an effort level of 1–2, increase the number of reps to 12–15 at the same resistance.

↓

When this becomes an effort level of 1–2, progress to the intermediate exercise. Establish a baseline at a resistance where you can complete 8–10 reps at an effort level of 4–5 and follow steps 2 through 4 before you move to the advanced exercise.

Confused? If you are a first-time exerciser, this may be a lot of information for you to process all at once. I can't stress enough how important it is to progress and challenge the skeletal muscles in different ways. Below is an example of the steps you would work through with respect to the chest muscles over a period of time. First, turn to the next chapter and locate chest muscle exercises (page 136). There are only two exercises for the chest—beginner and intermediate. Let's start at the beginning.

1. Go through your **warm-up** routine to get the muscles ready for your resistance training program.

2. The beginner exercise for chest is "Wall Push-ups," which you will start with. Start with the feet a few inches away from the wall and place the hands on the wall. Complete 8–10 reps and ask yourself: "What effort level would I say that was?" If your effort level was 4–5 then this is your baseline. If the exercise was too easy (level 1–2), then walk your feet a few inches away from the wall until the effort level becomes 4–5 at 8–10 reps. Do this exercise at this level for two to three weeks (2–3 times a week).

3. After two to three weeks, this particular exercise (at this level) should have reached an effort level of 1–2. It's time to progress. Look at step 4 in the progression chart, which instructs you to increase the reps to 12–15. So you will do the same exercise for another two to three weeks, completing 12–15 reps. You're getting stronger!

4. It's time to progress again. This time, the progression chart says to increase the resistance. Well, for this body part at beginner level, increasing the resistance means putting the **stability ball** (see page 94 for description of exercise equipment) between the wall and your hands. This is not what you might consider "increasing the resistance" but, in fact, adding the ball increases instability, increasing the load on the muscle fibers. Place your feet farther away from the wall until you can complete 8–10 reps at an effort level of 4–5. Making sense? It is all about finding a level that challenges *you* with a little guidance from your personal trainer, me! Continue at this level for two to three weeks.

5. The next progression, as the chart states, is another increase in repetitions. So continue this same exercise, doing 12–15 reps now for another couple of weeks.

6.   Now it's time to progress to the next exercise (intermediate). The intermediate exercise is "open and close on the ball." Again, you will start this at a resistance that is an effort level of 4–5 (this may mean doing it without any weights to start) and doing 8–10 reps.

7.   After a couple of weeks, increase the reps to 12–15 and continue until the effort level decreases to 1–2. Then increase the resistance (which means heavier weights for this particular exercise) a couple of pounds until the effort level is 4–5 at 8–10 reps. Then increase the reps again after a few weeks to 12–15.

Remember that "increasing resistance" can include: increasing the weights, moving hands down the band to another line, adding another piece of equipment or simply changing your body position. For some of you, a two-to-three-week progression period may be too long for some levels. This time frame is simply a guideline to ensure safety. Because every exercise is different, with some being more challenging than others, progression will occur at different times for different exercises. This is why keeping an **exercise log** (see page 98) is important. You have to read all the directions each time, and concentrate on what you feel and how much effort you put out.

Investing in Exercise

You'll need to make a small investment in equipment in order to implement the exercise program in this book. Fifteen years in the fitness business has exposed me to many workout gadgets, some great and some that are a waste of money. I've come up with suggestions for a few essentials that will cost you from $60 to $100—a small investment for a lifetime of stronger bones. All the necessary equipment can be purchased at fitness stores, department stores, health clinics and some drugstores. For some exercises, all you'll need is a sturdy chair, a towel, a bottom stair and a wall—no purchases necessary.

Stability Ball

The stability ball is an indispensable piece of equipment. It is a great tool for improving balance and core body strength and is used in balance exercises and as a bench or chair for resistance training exercises.

A stability ball is a big plastic ball filled with air. It comes in different sizes and colors and can be easily filled with a bicycle pump. When shopping for the correct size be sure to let the salesperson know your height. You should also try sitting on a filled ball in the store. Your thighs should be parallel to the floor with a 90 degree angle at your hips and knees. **For additional purchasing and safety tips, please refer to Appendix 2 (page 200).**

Weights or Dumbbells

I discourage you from purchasing weights that have removable ends that you must screw on and off to change the resistance. They may be more cost-effective but it is cumbersome to keep changing the ends during your workout. Individual dumbbells should be purchased at 3, 5, 8 and 10 lb. The weights will be used strictly for resistance-training exercises.

Exercise Band

An exercise band is a wide rubber elastic band that looks like a ribbon. The different colors it comes in represent different thicknesses and therefore different resistances. Purchase a medium-resistance band approximately 5 feet long, and draw horizontal lines across it with a marker, from the ends every 3 inches. Number the lines as shown below. This band should only cost you a few dollars and will also be used for resistance-training exercises.

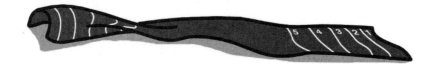

Supportive Shoes

You will need a pair of athletic shoes with a good sole. Running, walking or cross-trainer shoes will work fine. You don't need to spend a fortune, but the exercise footwear must be comfortable and supportive. You will need these especially for the weight-bearing or impact exercises described in Chapter 7.

Motivating Yourself

Getting started on an exercise program is, for some people, an easy task; staying on track, however, is often the hardest part. Here are a number of tips to keep you motivated and to keep you on track.

Schedule exercise appointments. Plan out your workout schedule on your calendar. Scheduling exercise appointments ensures that you've put aside enough time to fit in all the necessary components of the program. Make a shopping list of all the equipment you'll need. If you make a few phone calls before you head out shopping to ensure that the store has what you need, you can save a lot of time.

Keep an exercise log. Create an exercise log or journal that charts intensity, frequency, progressions, setbacks and goals. Use the journal to record the date and time of your workouts, the exercises you completed and how you felt both during and after your workout. Looking back through this log from time to time will give you a feeling of accomplishment and will motivate you to keep going. Write in your exercise journal even on the days you don't exercise, expressing how you feel that day and why you don't feel up to exercising. This practice will help you recognize your low-energy days and assist you in planning a more successful training schedule.

Work out with a buddy. Planning a workout with a friend is simply making an appointment that is difficult to cancel. An exercise partner can help you stick to your schedule, motivate you and help make the time go by quickly.

Divide the program into parts. Not everyone can devote one full hour a day to an exercise program. Divide the program into shorter segments throughout the day; you will be more likely to initiate a 15-minute session than a one-hour session. As long as two sets of each exercise are completed in one session, you can complete your program in as many small segments as you like.

Hire a personal trainer. Hiring a personal trainer is not necessary, but it is an extremely effective way to stick to your goals. This professional can check your form, motivate you to push yourself, consult on nutrition and other fitness information and simply knock on your door a few times a month to keep you going. If you decide to hire a personal trainer, check the individual's educational background and accreditations. A degree in the sciences is recommended but not essential. Certification through one of the many personal trainer programs is a must. Ask the trainer to give you a free consultation so that you can discuss your individual needs as they relate to osteoporosis.

Put on music. We all have particular songs that really get us moving. Put your favorite songs on a tape and play it while you exercise to keep you moving and motivated.

Keep your equipment where you can see it. Have you heard the phrase "out of sight, out of mind"? Keeping your exercise equipment in a place that is out of the way but easily seen will remind you to do your exercises daily. Moreover, pick an area in your home where you can comfortably do your exercises.

Planning Your Workout Schedule

Chapter 7 consists of five parts: warm-up, resistance training, weight bearing, balance-stability and stretching. To effectively plan your workout sessions, you must first know how much time each section requires and how you can manipulate particular parts to accommodate your schedule. The warm-up must always be done to ready the muscles and joints for demanding activities and to prevent injuries. The resistance-training part will be divided into sections A and B to ensure that related muscle groups are worked at different times and to make it easier to plan your workout time. This does not mean that the resistance-training sections A and B cannot be done all at once, if done in the order suggested here.

See the tables that follow for time requirements needed and for sample workout plans that will help you to organize your calendar.

Knowing If Your Body Is Ready

The exercises recommended in this book are safe for nearly everyone. However, it is always best to check with your doctor before increasing your physical activity particularly if you are over 69 years old or if you have osteoporosis or your risk for fracture is high. Before you start, answer these questions:

Yes No

❑ ❑ Do you have a heart condition and have been advised to only participate in physical activity recommended by a doctor?

❑ ❑ Do you feel chest pain or discomfort during physical activity or while you are resting?

❑ ❑ Do you become dizzy and lose your balance or lose consciousness?

❑ ❑ Do you have a bone or joint problem that could worsen as a result of physical activity?

❑ ❑ Are you are taking medication for your blood pressure or heart condition?

❑ ❑ Have you have experienced unexplained weight loss in the past six months?

If you answered yes to any of the above questions, you should talk to your doctor by phone or in person before starting these exercises.

The Bare Bones

- Proper progression is the most fundamental concept for the success of your exercise program. It ensures continual stress on the skeleton, which is needed for bone strength. Progression also eliminates boredom, decreases the occurrence of injuries and establishes goals to work towards.

- Implement progression, slowly increasing intensity by boosting the resistance, increasing the repetitions or advancing to the next exercise.

- Measuring your own physical effort requires you to determine how a particular exercise feels while you are doing it and how it feels at the end of the set. Assign a 1–2 effort level to a movement that challenges you minimally, and assign 4–5 to a movement that is very challenging to complete by the end of the set.

- You'll need to make a small investment in some exercise equipment. Purchase a stability ball that fits your individual height, and buy some weights or dumbbells, an exercise band and supportive non-slip shoes.

- Start an exercise journal that tracks the frequency, intensity, progressions and schedule of your workouts. This will help you stay focused and organized while working towards your goals.

- Check with your doctor either by phone or in person before making this program part of your weekly routine especially if you have osteoporosis or have not had a checkup in over a year.

seven

The Program

When my doctor told me to start an exercise program to help strengthen my bones, I asked her what exercises I should do. When she said, "resistance training and weight bearing," I was embarrassed to admit that I still didn't know what to do specifically.

—Lucy Riopell, personal training client

Congratulations! You've reached the part of the book where you can put into action all of the information you've learned about outwitting the Silent Thief with exercise. The exercises contained in this chapter have been developed to strengthen all of the individual muscle groups in your body, while they help you to improve your balance, stability and flexibility.

Read the "common mistakes" section of each exercise description whenever you perform the exercise. It is important to avoid forming bad habits in your technique, because repeating bad form can lead to injuries and, possibly, fractures.

This chapter provides you with warm-up, resistance and weight-bearing exercises; it also contains balance-stability drills and stretches. These exercises will challenge your body, keep you motivated and, most importantly, strengthen your bones to fight osteoporosis.

The Warm-Up

The purpose of the warm-up is to prepare the body—muscles and joints in particular—for exercise and the stresses placed upon them. Resistance-training and impact exercises load and lengthen the muscles and joints beyond their normal range, making warm-up exercises important in preventing injury and muscle strain. Warming up lubricates the joints and brings blood to the muscles for contraction readiness.

A warm-up should last 5–7 minutes and should incorporate nonstressful movements for all parts of the body. If you own a piece of cardio equipment, like a treadmill or stationary bike, use it for 5–7 minutes to warm up. (A brisk walk around the block, swinging the arms, will also do the job.) If you don't have access to this equipment, warm up the body by following the few simple movements listed in the table that follows (upper and lower body should be done together).

LOWER BODY	UPPER BODY
• March on the spot with high knees	• Circle arms in front of the body
• Side-step two steps to right then back to left	• Straight arms out to the side to shoulder height
• Alternate heel tap on floor, in front of body	• Press hands from shoulders out straight from chest
• Bend and straighten knees, feet shoulder-width apart	• Shrug the shoulders up towards the ears
• Alternate toe tap on floor behind the body	• Reach both arms up over the head

At the end of your warm-up, your body temperature should be elevated. In other words, you should be warm! Make your movements as big as you can, using the large muscle groups of the body (quadraceps, hamstrings, chest and back) for this routine.

Resistance Training

The resistance-training exercises described here are designed to challenge individual muscle groups. This part has been divided into section A and section B to make your workout schedule more flexible. The exercises in both sections A and B can be done on different days or all at once on one day. If time is an issue, the individual sections can be broken up throughout the day, with only one rule: you must always do two sets of each exercise during one exercise workout. For example, if you only have 15 free minutes for resistance training, do three exercises two times (two sets) each, *not* six different exercises one time (one set). Note: All references to "the ball" mean the stability ball (see page 94), and to "the band" mean the exercise band (see page 94).

Before you begin each exercise, take a deep breath, and as you slowly exhale, drop the shoulders down into the body, pull your chin in, bend your knees slightly and hold your tummy in tight.

TIME REQUIREMENTS OF WORKOUT

EXERCISE	FREQUENCY	DURATION	SETS	REPS
Warm-up	every workout	5 min	–	–
Resistance training	3 times/wk	A–20 min	2	8–15
		B–20 min	2	8–15
Weight-bearing	2 times/wk	15 min	2	8–30
Balance-training	1 time/wk	15 min	1	8–15
Stretching	3 times/wk	10 min	–	–

Sample Workout Plans

Pick a workout that fits your schedule. You can choose shorter daily workouts or exercise four times a week for a longer period. Resistance training has been divided into sections A and B to ensure that related muscle groups are worked at different times. However, both sections can be scheduled in the same workout with adequate rest between workout days.

Daily workout

EXERCISE	MON	TUES	WED	THU	FRI	SAT or SUN
Warm-up (5 min)	✓	✓	✓	✓	✓	✓
Resistance training - A&B (40 min)	A&B	–	A&B	–	A&B	–
Weight bearing (15 min)	–	✓	–	–	–	✓
Balance-training (15 min)	–	–	–	✓	–	–
Stretching (10 min)	–	✓	–	✓	–	✓
Duration in minutes	45	30	45	30	45	30

Four times per week

EXERCISE	MON	TUES	WED	THU	FRI	SAT or SUN
Warm-up (5 min)	✓	✓	off	✓	off	✓
Resistance training – A or B (20 min)	A	B	–	A	–	A&B
Weight bearing (15 min)	✓	–	–	✓	–	–
Balance-training (15 min)	–	✓	–	–	–	–
Stretching (10 min)	✓	✓	–	✓	–	–
Duration in minutes	50	50	–	50	–	45

THE EXERCISES

Warm-up 5 to 7 minutes (page 100)

Resistance training Section A (page 104–139)

MUSCLE GROUP	BEGINNER (●)	INTERMEDIATE (●●)	ADVANCED(●●●)
Biceps	Seated Hammer Curl	Standing Band Curl	
Quadriceps	Seated Leg Extension	Side Wall Press & Drop	Ball Squats
Medial Deltoid	Overhead Military Press	Diagonal Plane Shoulder Lift	
Wrist	Gather the Band	Roll the Weight	
Rhomboids	Wall Walk	Seated Shoulder Blade Squeeze	Ball Shoulder Blade Squeeze
Hamstrings	Standing Leg Curl	Ball Hamstring Dig & Roll	
Posterior Deltoid	Standing Shoulder Ball Press	Lying Shoulder Lift	
Chest	Wall Push-ups	Chest Open & Close on a Ball	

Resistance training Section B (page 140–173)

MUSCLE GROUP	BEGINNER (●)	INTERMEDIATE (●●)	ADVANCED(●●●)
Rotator Cuff	Closed Rotation with Band	Open Rotation with Band	
Neck	Ball Neck Press		
Hips	Seated Outer Press	Standing Ball Hip Press	Bend and Twist
Anterior Deltoid	Lying-down Band Pull	Top Half Lift	
Lower Back	Horse Stance	Ball Back Extensions	
Triceps	Seated Band Extension	Lying-down Band Press	
Calf	Standing Toe Press		
Lats	Seated Lat Pull	Lying-down Lat Pull	
Abdominals	Belly Button Press	Oblique Side Bends	

Weight-bearing or Impact Exercises (pages 175–179)

	BEGINNER (●)	INTERMEDIATE (●●)	ADVANCED(●●●)
	Modified Jumping Jack	Side Leap	One-footed North-South
	Sky Jump	Forward and Back Sky Jump	East-West Jump

Balance-training Exercises (pages 180–185)

	BEGINNER (●)	INTERMEDIATE (●●)	ADVANCED(●●●)
	Tandem Stance	Ball Leg Extension	One-legged Tabletop
	Stork Stance	Standing Toe Lift	

Stretching (pages 186–189)

Standing Chest Stretch
Quad and Hip Flexor Stretch
Hamstring Stretch
Spine and Abdominal Stretch (advanced)

Biceps (front upper arm) • beginner
Seated Hammer Curl

Body Position

Sit on the ball with feet flat on the floor, spine straight and tall, with arms hanging down by your sides. Weights are in your hands, with the ends of the dumbbells facing forward.

Exercise

Bend at the elbows and curl the weights up towards the shoulders, stopping two-thirds of the way up. Count 1-2-3 on the way up and the same on the way down. Always return the weights to a full hanging position. Keep the elbows tight to the side of the body and shoulders relaxed.

Always exhale during the exertion part of the exercise to keep your blood pressure from elevating too high. The exertion part of the exercise is the hardest part, as this is usually when the band is being stretched or your body or the weight are working against gravity.

Common Mistakes

Elbows travel forward on the curl, weights are brought up too high, or body sways forward and back to assist in the lifting of the weights.

Progression

1) Increase reps to 12–15

2) Increase the resistance by 2–3 pounds and decrease reps to 8–10

3) Increase reps to 12–15

4) Move to intermediate exercise.

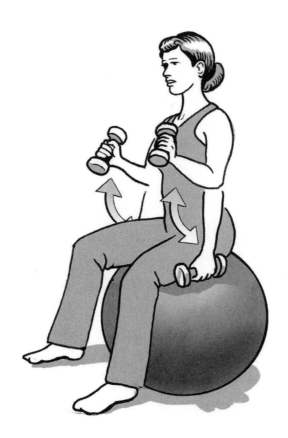

Biceps •• intermediate
Standing Band Curl

Body Position

Stand with foot on the middle of the band and hold ends in the hands. Stand tall with shoulders back and knees slightly bent.

Exercise

With the elbows tight to the side of the body, curl hands two-thirds of the way up and return to full hanging position. Count 1-2-3 on the way up and the same on the way down.

When lifting dumbbells or working with the band, do the exercise slowly so as not to strain the joints or use momentum to complete the task. Count slowly to three during the contraction phase and slowly to three during the lengthening phase of the movement. Remember, slower is better!

Common Mistakes

Again, elbows travel forward and away from the body on the curl, shoulders travel up towards the ears on the curl, or body sways back and forward to assist the curl.

Progression

1) Increase reps to 12–15
2) Increase the resistance by moving the hands down the band to another marked line and decrease reps to 8–10
3) Increase the reps to 12–15.

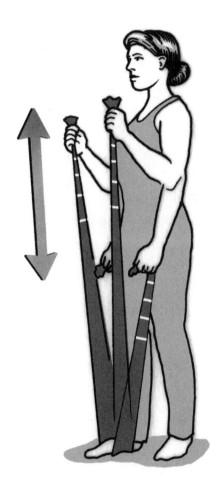

Quadriceps (front of thigh) • beginner
Seated Leg Extension

Body Position

Sit on the floor with your back up against a wall and buttocks close up to the wall. Both legs should be extended straight out from the body, side by side, with a rolled-up towel under the kneecap of the leg that you are about to work.

Exercise

The towel that is under the knee should create a slight bend in the knee of the working leg. Keep the upper back and shoulders against the wall and straighten the knee, pressing the back of the knee down into the towel. Hold the squeeze for a few seconds before releasing.

Common Mistakes

Shoulders round forward or whole body tenses up on the squeeze.

Progression

1) Increase reps to 12–15
2) Increase resistance by rolling up two towels (making a larger roll) and put them under the knee and decrease reps to 8–10
3) Increase reps to 12–15
4) Move to the intermediate exercise.

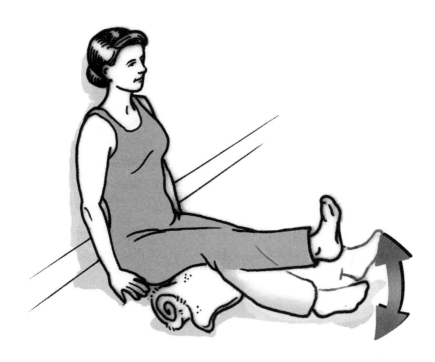

Quadriceps •• intermediate
Side Wall Press and Drop

Body Position

Stand sideways at a wall with the ball between your inside knee and the wall. Place the inside hand on the wall for balance and stand tall, with the tummy tight and shoulders back. Bend the inside foot back toward your buttocks so that your knee is on the ball. Tuck buttocks slightly under.

Exercise

There are two things going on at once in this exercise. First, press the inside knee sideways into the ball (into the wall). Second, while you do this, bend the outside knee (supporting leg), dropping the body down a few inches. You must keep pressing the inside knee against the ball on the drop.

Common Mistakes

Release of pressure of the knee into the ball, not keeping the back straight, or rolling forward on the toe on the bend.

Progression

1) Increase reps to 12–15
2) Remove hand from wall and decrease reps to 8–10
3) Increase reps to 15–20
4) Move to the advanced exercise.

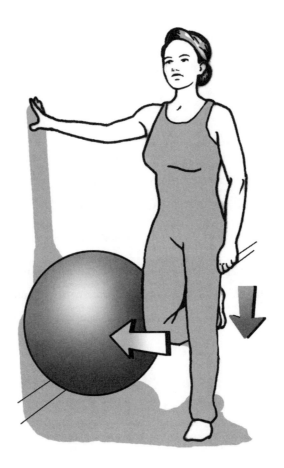

Quadriceps ●●● advanced
Ball Squats

Body Position

Stand and face away from the wall and put the ball between your tailbone and the wall. Place your feet about 4 feet out from the wall and lean back into the ball.

Exercise

Sit down into an imaginary chair, dropping the buttocks as low as you can. As you sit, let the ball roll up the back, push through your heels and always keep the knees behind the toes. Keep the shoulders back and pressed into the ball on the squat. Roll the tailbone under the ball on the drop.

Common Mistakes

Upper back comes away from the ball or knees travel out over the toes on the squat. Feet must be placed at a distance far out from the wall to start.

Progression

1) Increase reps to 12–15
2) Increase resistance by performing the squats on one leg only, hold the other leg out front and decrease the reps to 8–10
3) Increase reps to 12–15.

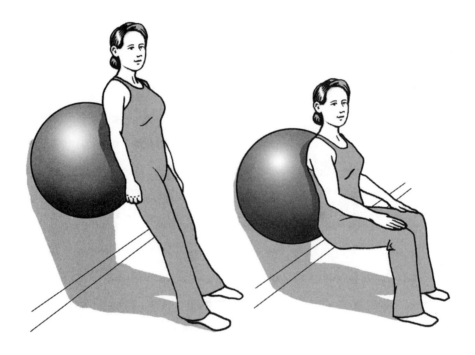

Medial Deltoid (middle shoulder) • beginner
Overhead Military Press

Body Position

Sit on the ball with your feet flat on the floor, spine straight and tall and arms in a "W" shape (elbows out the side and hands up). Weights are in your hands with your palms facing forward and elbows are out to the side but slightly in front of the line of the body (very important).

Exercise

I sometimes call this the "A" and "W" press because your arms form the shapes of the those letters at the beginning and the end of the movement. Begin with arms in "W" shape with the elbows and weights slightly in front of the body and press arms up straight over the head to "A" shape. At the top, the weights should also be slightly in front of the body and arms straight. Return down to "W" shape.

Common Mistakes

Elbows are back behind the body, arms do not travel all the way up until they are straight, or weights come too close to the body during the lowering phase.

Progression

1) Increase reps to 12–15
2) Increase the resistance by 2–3 pounds and decrease reps to 8–10
3) Increase reps to 12–15
4) Move to the intermediate exercise.

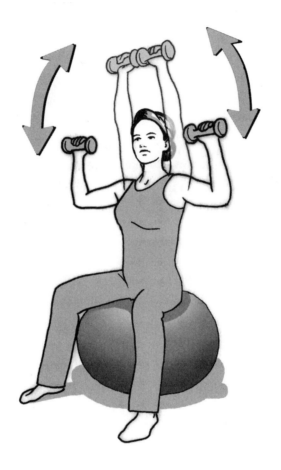

Medial Deltoid •• intermediate
Diagonal Plane Shoulder Lift

Body Position

Lie sideways over the ball, with the ball under the hip and hand over the ball on the floor for balance. Keep the body straight and shoulders high. The weight is in the top hand and the arm is straight along the line of the body.

Exercise

Start with the arm straight down the line of the body, slightly lower than the top knee. Lift straight arm up until it is parallel with the floor (this is not a very big range) and return back to top knee.

Common Mistakes

Support shoulder rides up during the exercise or weight is lifted too high.

Progression

1) Increase reps to 12–15
2) Move ball up under the armpit so that you must support your own body weight from shoulder to feet and decrease reps to 8–10
3) Increase reps to 12–15.

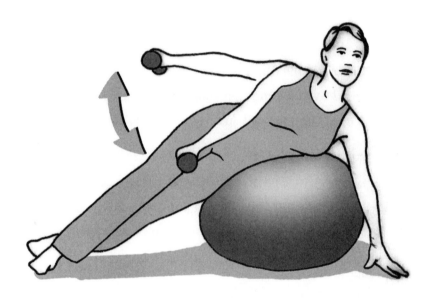

Wrist • beginner
Gather the Band

Stand or sit with tummy tucked in and spine tall. Hold hand out in front of the body with one end of the band in the palm, which is facing down.

Exercise

Gather the band up in the fist, using the palm and fingers without rotating the wrist. When the whole band is in your hand or you can't grasp any more of it, let it go, hang on to the end and repeat. Do both arms.

Common Mistakes

Using only the thumb or only the fingers to do the gathering. Be sure to use both. Don't rotate the wrist while gathering.

Progression

1) Increase reps to 12–15
2) Increase sets to 3 and decrease reps to 8–10
3) Increase reps to 12–15
4) Progress to the intermediate exercise.

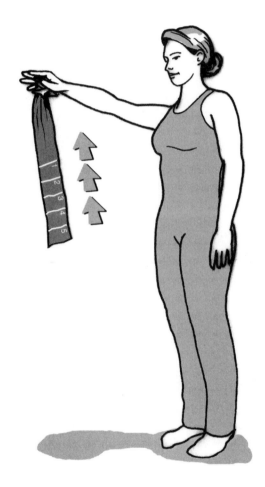

Wrist •• intermediate
Roll the Weight

Body Position

Stand or sit with tummy tucked in and spine tall. Hold both hands out in front with palms around the ends of the dumbbell.

Exercise

Hold your hands out in front of the body and roll the weight toward you in your hands, alternating left- and right-hand roll. On the second set, roll the weight away from you. Only move the wrist, not the elbows or shoulders.

Common Mistakes

Moving the elbows and shoulders during the roll.

Progression

1) Increase reps to 12–15
2) Increase the weight by 2–3 pounds and decrease reps to 8–10
3) Increase reps to 12–15.

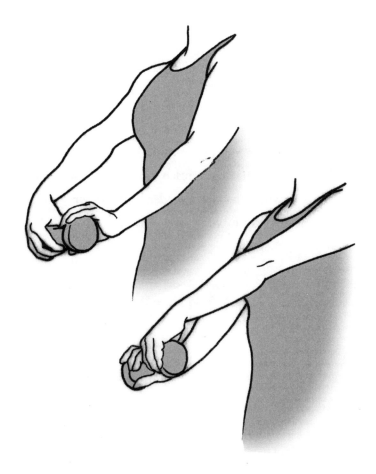

Rhomboids (muscles between shoulder blades)
• beginner
Wall Walk

Body Position

Stand tall, and face the wall, about one foot away from it. Place your fingertips on the wall, just above shoulder level.

Exercise

Walk your fingertips up the wall (like a spider) as high as you can. Let the shoulder blades rise up as your fingers reach the top of the walk. As you walk the fingertips back down, bring the shoulder blades down also. Keep your weight back in your feet, not forward into the wall.

> Holding your tummy in tight, especially during the standing exercises, will stabilize the pelvic region, thereby protecting the lower back.

Progression

1) Increase reps to 12–15
2) Move the feet in, standing as close to the wall as possible and decrease reps to 8–10
3) Increase reps to 12–15
4) Progress to the intermediate exercise.

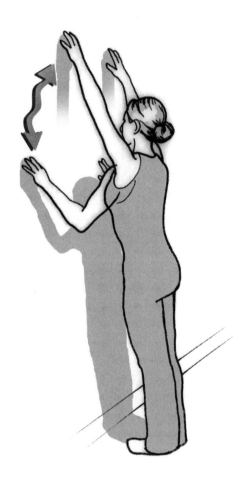

Rhomboids ●● intermediate
Seated Shoulder Blade Squeeze

Body Position

Sit in a chair with your feet flat on the floor and your spine up against the back of the chair. Lift your elbows out to the side to just 1 inch below shoulder height with the hands forward.

Exercise

Slowly bring the elbows back, behind the line of the body, squeezing the shoulder blades together and sticking out the chest. Think of cracking an imaginary egg between the shoulder blades. Remember that the shoulder blades must come together for this exercise to work.

Common Mistakes

Elbows come back without the shoulder blades coming together.

Progression

1) Increase reps to 12–15
2) Add the band. Extend one leg straight and wrap the middle of the band around the foot with the ends in the hands. Repeat the above movement for 8–10 reps
3) Increase reps to 12–15
4) Progress to the advanced exercise.

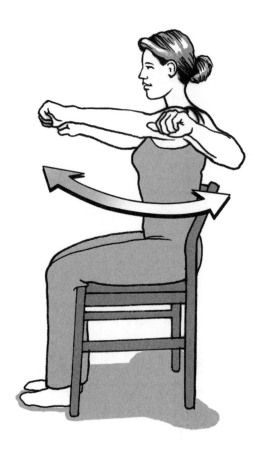

Rhomboids ●●● advanced
Ball Shoulder Blade Squeeze

Body Position

Lie forward over the ball with it under the lower chest and ribcage. Keep your toes on the floor behind you for balance. Keep head straight in a neutral position so as not to stress the neck. Arms are in the same position as the intermediate exercise.

Exercise

With the weights in your hands, bring the elbows back and around the body, squeezing the shoulder blades together, pressing the chest into the ball. Crack that egg! Do not rest the weights on the floor between lifts.

Common Mistakes

Shoulder blades not coming fully together.

Progression

1) Increase reps to 12–15
2) Increase the resistance by 2–3 pounds and decrease the reps to 8–10
3) Increase the reps to 12–15.

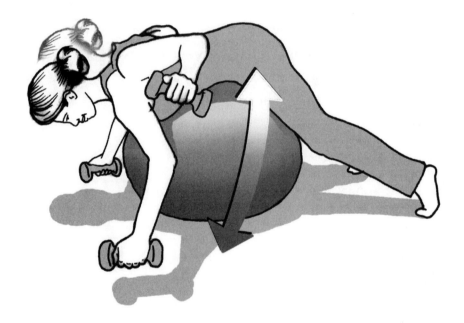

Hamstrings (back of thigh) • beginner
Standing Leg Curl

Body Position

Face the wall, 6 inches away, with hands on the wall for balance. Body weight is on the nonworking leg to free up the other one.

Exercise

Make a loop out of the band by tying a knot in it. Make the loop about 8 inches across. If working the right hamstring, put the right foot through the loop and *stand* on the other side of the loop with the left foot. Flex the right foot (toes towards the knee) and curl the right heel back towards the buttocks, pulling on the band. Your foot will only travel about halfway up. Switch legs. Keep both knees lined up, side by side, during the exercise.

Common Mistakes

Knee of the working leg travels back during the curl.

Progression

1) Increase reps to 12–15
2) Walk the feet about 6 more inches away from the wall and bend the torso about 30 degrees forward (bending at the hips). Hands are still on the wall for support. Decrease reps to 8–10
3) Increase reps to 12–15
4) Progress to the intermediate exercise.

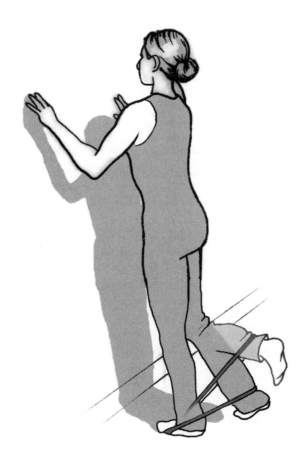

Hamstrings •• intermediate
Ball Hamstring Dig and Roll

Body Position

Lie flat on your back on the floor with your heels resting up on top of the ball. Extend the arms out to the side along the floor and lift the pelvis slightly off the floor.

Exercise

Dig the heels into the ball and roll it toward the buttocks, keeping the pelvis off the floor and tucking the butt under (pelvic tilt). Extend the legs back out, rolling the ball away from the body. Keep the pelvis elevated at all times and toes pointed up to the ceiling. Small rolls are better.

Common Mistakes

Ball is rolled in too much or pelvis is lifted too high off the ground.

Progression

1) Increase reps to 12–15
2) Perform the same exercise with only one leg. The other leg is extended straight up in the air. This version is very advanced, progress to this one slowly!
3) Increase reps to 12–15.

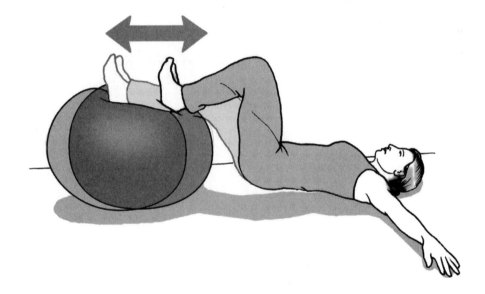

Posterior deltoid (back of the shoulder)
• beginner
Standing Shoulder Ball Press

Body Position

Stand sideways to the wall with the inside arm extended forward at shoulder height and the palm facing down. Place the ball between the extended wrist and the wall.

Exercise

Slowly press the side of the wrist into the ball and release. Keep the shoulder down on the press. This is a very small movement. Keep the spine tall and tummy tucked in.

Common Mistakes

Shoulder travels up on the arm press.

Progression

1) Increase reps to 12–15
2) Angle arm up about 8 inches with the ball along the wall. Arm is slightly above the head. Decrease reps to 8–10
3) Increase reps to 12–15
4) Progress to the intermediate exercise.

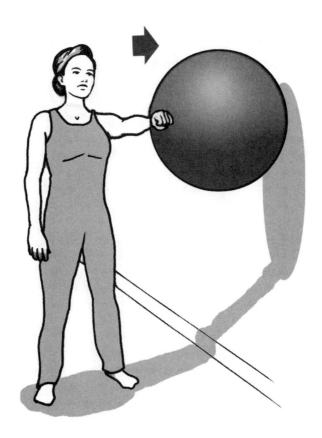

Posterior deltoid •• intermediate
Lying Shoulder Lift

Body Position

Lie on the floor on your side with the bottom arm tucked under the head. Bend the top knee and rest it on the floor in front of the body for support. Roll slightly forward and extend the top arm out along the floor at eye level.

Exercise

Hold the weight in the hand of the extended arm. Lift the weight 8–10 inches off the floor, keeping the arm straight and reaching from the shoulder on the lift. Do not rest the weight on the floor between lifts.

Common Mistakes

Body rolls back and forward on the lift. Weight is lifted too high.

Progression

1) Increase reps to 12–15
2) Increase resistance by 2–3 pounds and decrease reps to 8–10
3) Increase reps to 12–15.

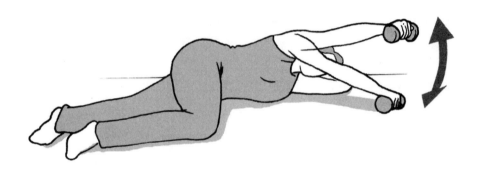

Chest • beginner
Wall Push-ups

Body Position

Stand and face the wall with your feet about 12 inches away from it. Place your hands on the wall at shoulder height, then slide them down a few inches. Keep your tummy tucked in and spine straight.

Exercise

Slowly bend the elbows, bringing the chest and upper body as close to the wall as you can. If you can't get the chest close, move the feet a little closer and start there. Slowly press the chest and body away until the arms are straight. Keep your heels on the floor at all times. Full body moves as one unit.

Common Mistakes

Chest moves close to the wall while the hips stay away (body not moving as one unit). Chest doesn't get close enough to the wall.

Progression

1) Increase reps to 12–15
2) Put the ball between the hands and the wall and move the feet farther away from the wall. Do push-ups as before and decrease the reps to 8–10
3) Increase reps to 12–15
4) Progress to the intermediate exercise.

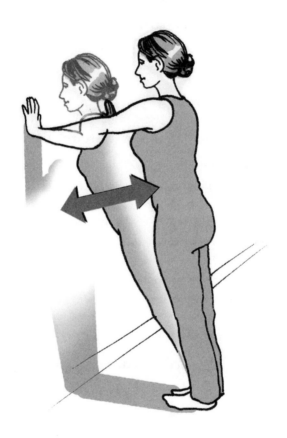

Chest •• intermediate
Chest Open and Close on Ball

Body Position

Start by sitting on the ball, walk your feet out and away from the ball, letting the ball roll up the back. With the weights in your hands at the chest, lean back into the ball and form a tabletop position. Rest the head on the ball and keep the hips high.

Exercise

Hold the weights side by side up over the chest with the arms straight. Open the arms, dropping the elbows below the line of the body. Arms form a "W" shape on the drop. Press the weights back up to straight arms over the chest.

Common Mistakes

Elbows don't bend enough on the drop. Arms do not return to straight line above the chest. Hips start to drop through the reps.

Progression

1) Increase reps to 12–15
2) Increase weight by 3–5 pounds and decrease reps to 8–10
3) Increase reps to 12–15.

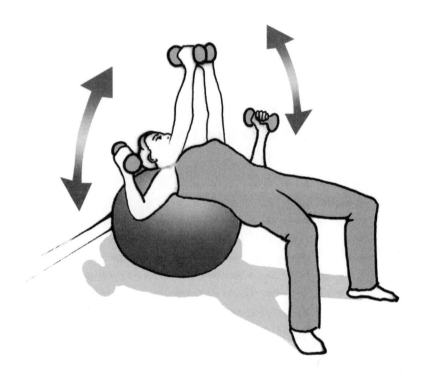

Rotator Cuff (shoulder) ● beginner
Closed Rotation with Band

Body Position

Sit on chair with your feet flat on the floor. To work the right rotator cuff, hold one end of the band in the left hand at the hip and the other in the right hand. Keep the right elbow tight to the waist with the arm bent at 90 degrees and the hand in front. There should be a little tension on the band in this position.

Exercise

Keeping the elbow tight to the body, stretch the band by opening the hand to the right, away from the body. Only open the arm as far as you can without the elbow coming away from the body.

Common Mistakes

Elbow comes away from the waist. Band doesn't start off tight enough at the beginning position.

Progression

1) Increase reps to 12–15
2) Move the hand down a line on the band to increase the resistance. Decrease reps to 8–10
3) Increase reps to 12–15
4) Progress to the intermediate exercise.

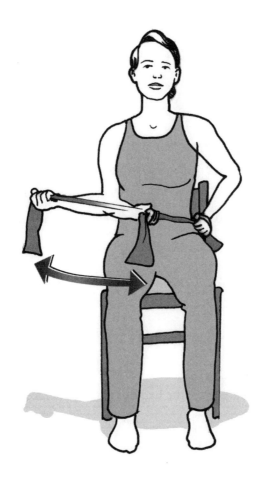

Rotator Cuff (shoulder) •• intermediate
Open Rotation with Band

Body Position

Same as the beginner exercise except the tension on the band at the start position is looser.

Exercise

Draw a diagonal line in space, moving the shoulder joint only, with the hand ending above the head and out to the side. Elbow comes away from the body as the arm travels out and up and ends up at shoulder height. Keep the spine pressed up against the back of the chair and shoulders down.

Common Mistakes

Shoulders rise up as the arm moves out and up. Elbow does not make it up to shoulder height.

Progression

1) Increase reps to 12–15
2) Move the hand down a line on the band to increase the resistance. Decrease reps to 8–10
3) Increase reps to 12–15.

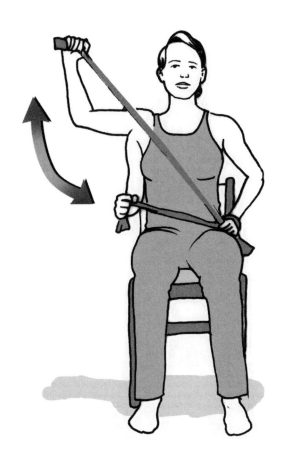

Neck • beginner and intermediate
Ball Neck Press

Body Position

Stand sideways to the wall with the ball between the side of the head (above the ear) and the wall. Stand tall with the shoulders down and tummy tucked in.

Exercise

Slowly and lightly press the head sideways into the ball and release. The press should come from above the ear—not the whole body. Work both sides.

Common Mistakes

Pressing too hard.

Progression

Turn the body and face the wall, with forehead on the ball, and press forward as the picture indicates.

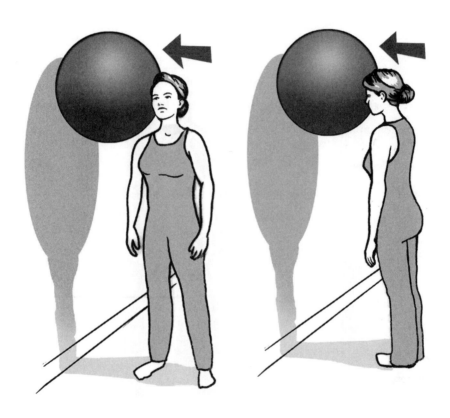

Hips • beginner
Seated Outer Press

Body Position

Sit on a chair, place the middle of the band under both feet, cross it and hold the ends of the band in the hands at the hips. Sit up tall.

Exercise

While holding the band at the hips, slowly open the legs, spreading the feet and knees apart and slowly bring them together. Keep the knees and toes in line on the open and close. Move the whole leg as one unit.

Common Mistakes

Feet open without the knees coming apart. Body leans forward during the exercise.

Progression

1) Increase reps to 12–15
2) Move the hands down the band a line to increase the resistance. Decrease reps to 8–10
3) Increase reps to 12–15
4) Progress to the intermediate exercise.

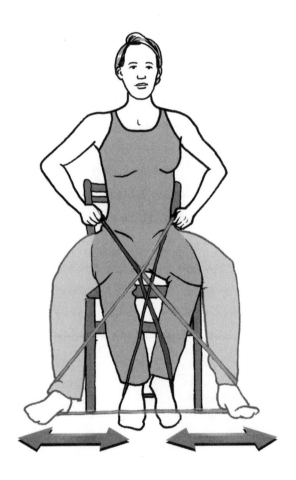

Hips •• intermediate
Standing Ball Hip Press

Body Position

Stand sideways to the wall, weight on the outside foot. Put the ball between the thigh of the inside leg and the wall. Keep the inside foot slightly off the floor and the knee in line with the outside knee. Place the inside hand on the wall for balance.

Exercise

Moving along a line parallel to the floor, slowly press the inside leg into the ball, into the wall, and slowly release. Keep the knee of the supporting leg slightly bent and the spine straight.

Common Mistakes

Inside hip rises up on the leg press.

Progression

1) Increase reps to 12–15
2) Move the ball and the inside leg slightly to the front of the body (about 6–8 inches) and repeat the exercise. Decrease reps to 8–10
3) Increase reps to 12–15
4) Progress to the advanced exercise.

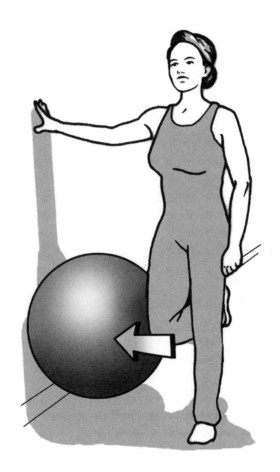

Hips ●●● advanced
Bend and Twist

Body Position

Stand sideways to the wall, right hip toward the wall, about 1 foot away from the wall. Place the right hand on the wall for balance and bend the left knee (outside leg) back 90 degrees. Line up the knees.

Exercise

Keeping the right hand on the wall for balance, bend the right knee, drop the buttocks and touch the left hand down to the outside of the right foot. Left foot stays bent back but knees stay lined up. Sit back into an imaginary chair. Press back up to standing position. Repeat on the left leg.

Common Mistakes

Bending at the back, not the knee and hip. Right knee must bend and buttocks must drop towards the floor. Left knee slides back on the bend— keep them side by side always.

Progression

1) Increase reps 12–15
2) Hold a 5 lb weight in the left hand while doing the exercise. Continue doing 12–15 reps
3) Increase reps to 15–20.

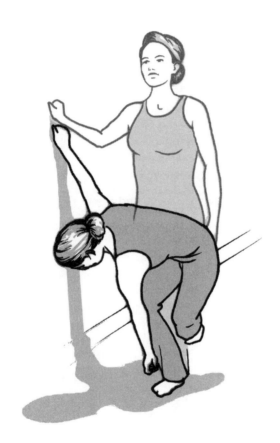

Anterior deltoid (front of shoulder)
• beginner
Lying-down Band Pull

Body Position

Lie on your back with the legs flat on the floor. Put the middle of the band around the soles of the feet, hold the ends with the hands and keep the arms straight down along the side of the body. If your band is short, you may bend the knees up with the feet flat on the floor and the middle of the band under them. There must be some tension on the band at start position.

Exercise

Lift the straight arms up over the body and right up above the head. Keep the arms straight and slowly lower them back down to the side of the body.

Common Mistakes

Elbows bend on the pull.

Progression

1) Increase reps to 12–15
2) Move the hands down a line to increase the resistance.
   Decrease reps to 8–10
3) Increase reps to 12–15
4) Progress to the intermediate exercise.

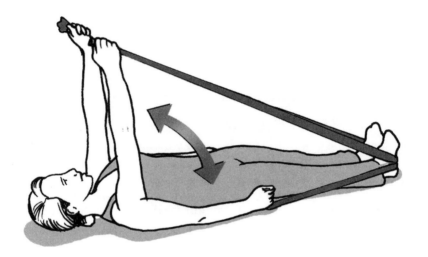

Anterior deltoid •• intermediate
Top Half Lift

Body Position

Lean your back up against the wall with the feet 6 inches away on the floor. Hold the weights in the hands with the ends of the dumbbells facing up, palms facing each other and arms extended straight out in front of the body at shoulder height.

Exercise

This is a difficult exercise; you may want to begin it without any weights. Starting with the arms extended straight out in front of the body at shoulder height, lift straight arms up above the head (slightly in front of the head) and return down to in front of the body. Keep your upper back against the wall.

Common Mistakes

Upper back comes away from the wall during the exercise. Arms do not stay straight on the lift.

Progression

1) Increase reps 12–15
2) Add weights or increase the resistance by 2–3 pounds and decrease reps to 8–10
3) Increase reps to 12–15.

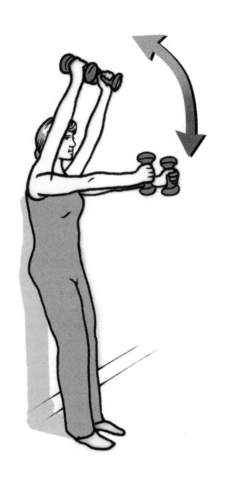

Lower back • beginner

Horse Stance

Body Position

Get onto your hands and knees with the hips directly over the knees and the shoulders directly over the hands. Keep the head straight (nose pointing to the floor).

Exercise

Slowly lift the right palm and the left knee slightly off the floor (just high enough to slide a magazine under the palm or knee). Lift alternating hands with the opposite knee and hold briefly at the elevated position for a few seconds.

Common Mistakes

Lifting the knee and hand too high while swaying side to side to accommodate the lift.

Progression

1) Increase reps to 12–15
2) Increase the resistance by lifting and then extending the arm and leg straight out, no higher than the height of the body. Decrease reps to 8–10
3) Increase reps to 12–15
4) Progress to the intermediate exercise.

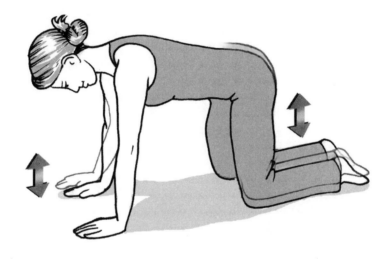

Lower back •• intermediate
Ball Back Extensions

Body Position

Lie forward over the ball with it under the tummy. Keep the legs bent and the toes on the floor. Place the hands behind the head with the elbows open.

Exercise

Press the hips into the ball and lift the torso slightly above the line of the body. Keep the elbows open wide and do not lift too high.

Common Mistakes

Elbows come together on the lift, torso comes up too high or body swings on the lift.

Progression

1) Increase reps to 12–15
2) Extend the arms out straight above the head and join the hands.
   Decrease reps to 8–10
3) Increase reps to 12–15.

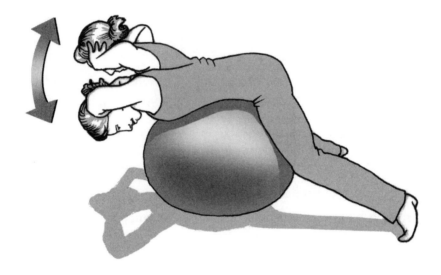

Triceps (back of upper arm) • beginner
Seated Band Extension

Body Position

Sit on the chair with the band draped over the right shoulder. Keep the spine straight and tall. Bend the right elbow 90 degrees and grab both ends of the band. The elbow should be slightly behind the line of the body and arm squeezed tight into your side. There should be some tension on the band in this position.

Exercise

Slowly straighten the arm, lengthening the band, pressing the hand down towards the floor. Keep the elbow back and arm tight into the body at all times. Go all the way down to a straight arm.

Common Mistakes

The elbow moves forward and back or the arm comes away from the body on the arm extension. Not enough tension on the band.

Progression

1) Increase reps to 12–15
2) Move the hand up the band to the next line to increase the resistance.
   Decrease reps to 8–10
3) Increase reps to 12–15
4) Progress to the intermediate exercise.

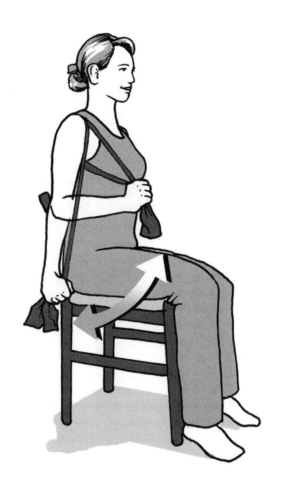

Triceps •• intermediate
Lying-down Band Press

Body Position

Lie flat on your back with your knees bent up. Put the band around behind the upper back and up under the armpits. You are lying on the band. Hold the ends of the band in your hands at ear level, with elbows pointed up towards the ceiling.

Exercise

Straighten the arms by extending the hands up towards the ceiling, stretching the band up. Bend the elbows, dropping the hands back down beside the ears. Keep the elbows in the same spot in space at all times.

Common Mistakes

Elbows travel toward the hips during the extension or arms don't get all the way up straight over the head. Make sure the shoulder joint does not move during this exercise.

Progression

1) Increase reps to 12–15
2) Slide the hands down the band one line to increase the resistance.
   Decrease reps to 8–10
3) Increase reps to 12–15.

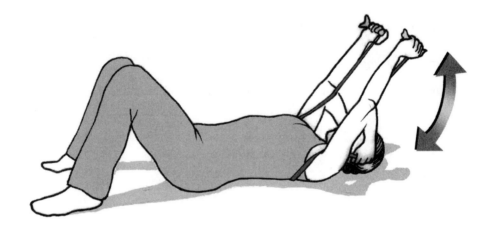

Calf • beginner and intermediate
Standing Toe Press

Body Position

Stand facing the wall with the feet 10–12 inches away from the wall. Place both hands on the wall for balance.

Exercise

Slowly elevate the whole body straight up on the toes as high as you can. If 8–10 reps of this is too easy, move the feet another 6 inches away from the wall. Do not rest the heels on the floor between lifts.

Common Mistakes

Rolling the foot out on the lift or resting on the heels between the lifts.

Progression

1) Increase reps to 12–15
2) Do the same exercise on one foot only. Decrease reps to 8–10
3) Increase reps to 12–15
4) Increase reps to 15–20.

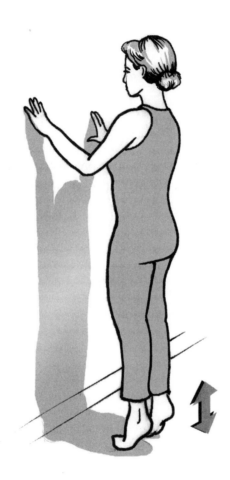

Lats (back) • beginner
Seated Lat Pull

Body Position

Sit on chair with feet flat on the floor and spine straight and tall. Hold the band in both hands, up, above and slightly in front of the head. Keep the shoulders and shoulder blades down during the exercise.

Exercise

Hold one side of the band tightly with one hand, keeping the arm straight. Pull the other half of the band down with one arm, bending the elbow down toward and past the side of the body. Do one arm entirely, then the other.

Common Mistakes

Shoulders and shoulder blades rise up during the exercise.

Progression

1) Increase reps to 12–15
2) Slide the hand up the band one line to increase the resistance. Decrease reps to 8–10
3) Increase reps to 12–15
4) Progress to the intermediate exercise.

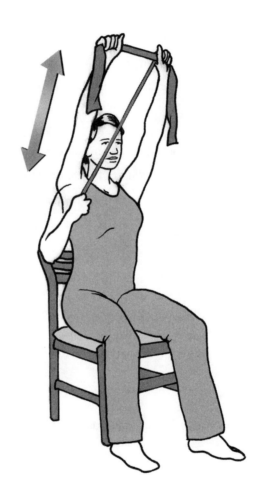

Lats •• intermediate
Lying-down Lat Pull

Body Position

Lie flat on your back with knees bent up and feet flat on the floor. Hold both weights together in both hands on the floor above the head. Arms are bent approximately 45 degrees at the elbows. Elbows are pointed up to the ceiling.

Exercise

Lift the weights off the floor and bring them up over the chest, keeping arms bent at the same angle. Press the shoulder blades down toward the lower back on the lift. Stop when the weights are over the chest and slowly return back over the head towards the floor. Only the shoulder joint moves during this exercise.

Common Mistakes

The angle at the elbow changes throughout the exercise. Arms don't reach all the way back over the head to the floor.

Progression

1) Increase reps to 12–15
2) Increase the resistance by 3–5 pounds total. Decrease reps to 8–10
3) Increase reps to 12–15.

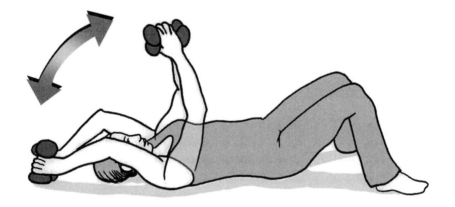

Abdominals • beginner
Belly Button Press

Body Position

Lie flat on your back with the knees bent up, feet flat on the floor and head also back on the floor. Hands rest on top of your tummy.

Exercise

Press your belly button down toward your spine and the floor. Hold it for 5 counts then release. As you pull in your belly button, press your lower back into the floor. Start with 10 reps.

Progression

1) Increase reps to 12–15
2) Place your hands behind your head and rest your head back in your hands. Lift your head and shoulders up as you press your belly button down. Decrease reps to 8–10
3) Increase reps to 12–15
4) Progress to the intermediate exercise.

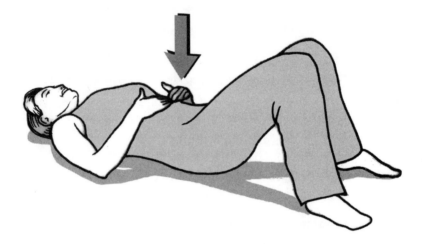

Abdominals •• intermediate
Oblique Side Bends

Body Position

Stand with your feet shoulder-width apart and the right hand hanging down by your side. Place the left hand behind the head with the elbow pressed back, and slightly bend the knees.

Exercise

Bend the torso over to the right side, letting the hand slide down the right leg and tipping the left elbow up towards the ceiling. Bend to the side as much as you can without leaning forward or sliding the hips to the left. Put most of your body weight on the right leg to stop the hips from sliding. You should feel this on the left side by the waist and ribs. Repeat on the other side.

Common Mistakes

Hips sliding to the opposite side from that which you are bending to, leaning forward on the side bend, and elbow not tipping up to the ceiling. Leaning forward during this exercise can put your spine at risk!

Progression

1) Increase the reps to 12–15
2) Increase the resistance by placing a 3–5 lb. weight in the hanging arm and decrease the reps to 8–10
3) Increase the reps to 12–15.

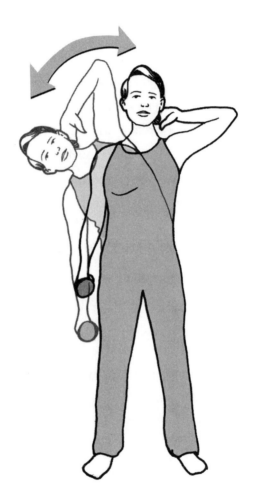

Weight–Bearing or Impact Exercises

In Chapter 5, you learned about the importance of impact exercises to bone health. Vertical jumping is the best high-impact exercise for building bone. These exercises should be reserved for the individual who is premenopausal and doesn't suffer from osteoporosis. If you have been diagnosed with osteopenia, consult your doctor before participating in the exercises described in this section. Remember that you must warm up for these exercises, as you did for the resistance-training exercises. You may do one, a few, or all of the following exercises during one workout or spread them out over a week or day. I suggest that you spread them out throughout your workout so as not to overstrain the knees and back. If you are doing the following exercises all at once, please take a two-minute break between them.

Important Jumping Information

You may jump on any flat surface that is not slippery. To prevent falls or collisions with walls or furniture, check the surface of the floor and the space allowance before beginning. Wear comfortable and supportive shoes—running shoes are best. *Always* start with the beginner impact exercises and progress to the intermediate; try advanced jumps only after doing the beginner ones for a few weeks. Any one of the following exercises will do the job!

Weight-bearing ● beginner

Modified Jumping Jack

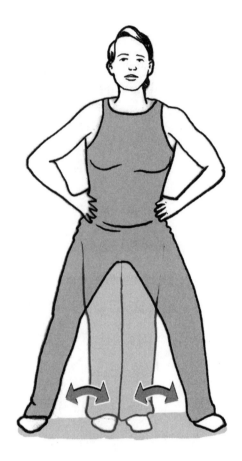

Stand tall with your feet together, side by side, knees slightly bent and hands on hips. Bend your knees, jump up, open your legs and land with your feet approximately shoulder-width apart. Land on the balls of your feet, then let heels down with a knee bend. Repeat the jump, bringing the feet together to start position. Start with 10 reps and then progress slowly to 20–30. A jump in and out constitutes one repetition.

Weight-bearing • beginner
Sky Jump

Stand tall with your feet a few inches apart, knees slightly bent and arms hanging down by your sides. Bend your knees and jump straight up, bringing the arms above the head, reaching for the sky. Land on the balls of your feet and bend the knees. Feet take off and land in the same spot. Start with 10 reps then progress slowly to 20–30.

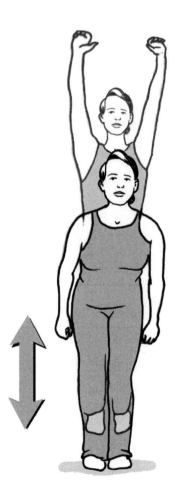

Weight-bearing •• intermediate
Side Leap

Stand on your left foot with the right foot elevated and your hands on hips. Bend your left knee and jump up and sideways to the right, landing on your right foot only. Jump sideways only 1–2 feet as high as you can. Repeat jump, starting on the right foot, jumping to the left and landing on the left foot. Start with 10 reps then progress slowly to 20–30.

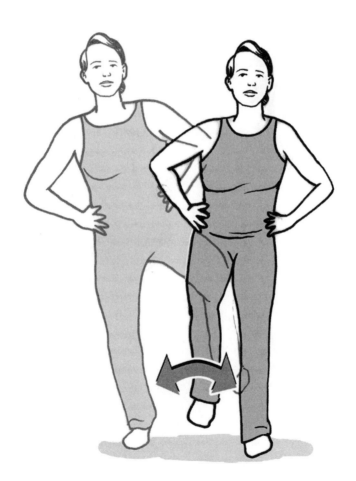

Weight-bearing •• intermediate

Forward and Back Sky Jump

This jump is exactly the same as the sky jump (page 176) except that you will travel forward and back with these jumps. Start with the feet a few inches apart, with your hands down by your sides. Bend your knees, jump up and forward about 1 foot, landing on the balls of your feet. Bend the knees on the landing. You will do 2 jumps forward followed by 2 jumps back. Start with 10 reps then progress to 15–20.

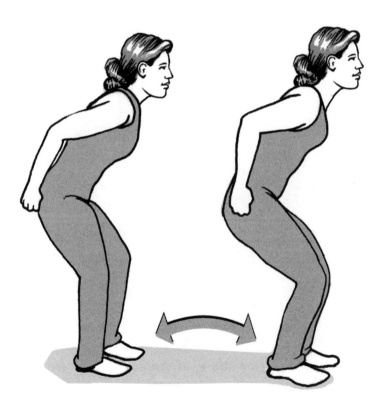

Weight-bearing ••• advanced
One-footed North-South-East-West Jump

Stand on one foot with the knee slightly bent and hands on hips. Make your starting position the center position and jump north (forward), landing on the same foot, then back to center position, again, landing on the same foot. Jump east (right) then back to center, jump south (back) then back to center and finally west (left) then back to center. Repeat on the other leg. Start with 8 reps (4, each leg) then progress to 12.

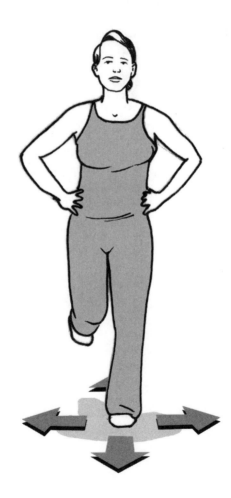

Balance-Training Exercises

Balance exercises do not directly strengthen the bones but are important in the prevention of falls leading to bone breaks or fractures. Practicing balance improves your stability while taxing your core muscles (abdominals, spine and pelvic muscles). They also strengthen the supporting muscles of the lower limb joints (ankles and knees) while exercising the brain. When you begin the balance exercises, you'll be surprised at how challenging they are.

Important Balance Information

Always perform balance exercises on a flat non-slippery floor wearing non-slip shoes—running shoes are best. You should have a wall, countertop or heavy piece of furniture close by to grab onto to prevent falling if your balance is compromised too much. Begin with the beginner exercises and progress to the intermediate and advanced ones as your balance improves. You measure balance improvement by your ability to maintain a position of the exercise for longer periods of time. Always do 2 sets of the exercise. Wobbling during the exercises is a sign that balance is being worked on. Wobbling is a good thing!

Balance-training • beginner

Tandem Stance

Stand with one foot in front of the other in a straight line (front heel at back toe) with arms out to the side. Maintain this position for 10 seconds. Progress by repeating this exercise with the eyes closed. Be sure that something is close by to grab onto in case you lose your balance.

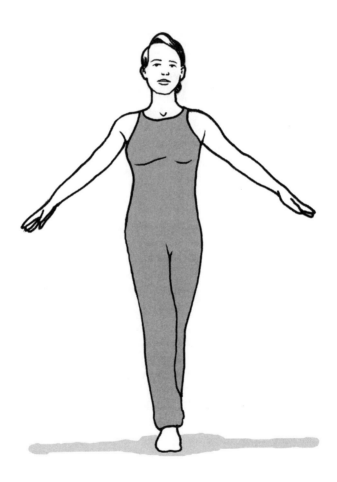

Balance-training ● beginner

Stork Stance

Stand on one foot with the other bent up at the supporting knee. With the arms extended to the side, hold this position for 10 seconds. Do this on the other foot. Progress by repeating this exercise with eyes closed.

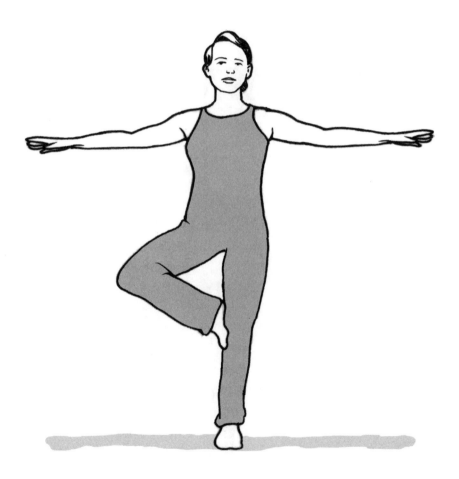

Balance-training •• intermediate
Ball Leg Extension

Sit on the ball with your buttocks on top, in the center, and feet flat on the
floor. Extend the arms to the side and slowly straighten out one leg at the
knee. Hold this position for 10 seconds then repeat on the other leg.
Progress by repeating this exercise with eyes closed.

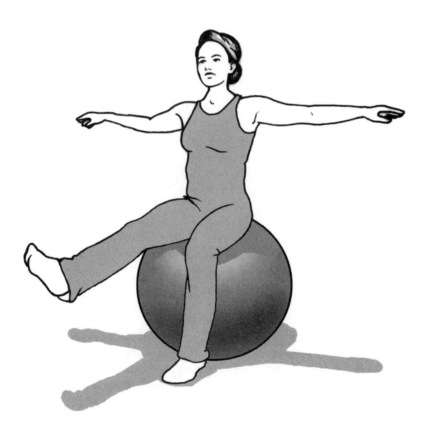

Balance-training •• intermediate
Standing Toe Lift

Stand on one foot with the other flat on top of the ball in front of the body.
Slowly lift the body up on the supporting toe as high as you can, bringing
both arms straight out to the side and then up over the head. Hold only 1–2
seconds then lower heel to the floor. Do 12 reps before switching legs.
Progress by holding the body up on your toe for 8 seconds before lowering.

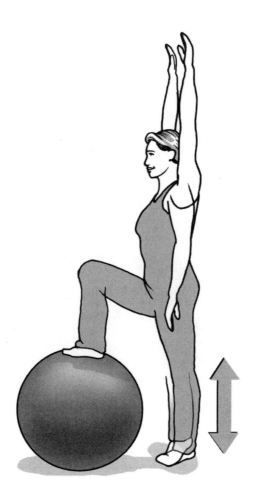

Balance-training ••• advanced
One-Legged Tabletop

Start by sitting on the ball, walk your feet out as you, lean back onto the ball and let it roll up the spine to a tabletop position. This movement alone takes practice. Take your time learning to get into this position. The ball should be under the head and neck, and the knees should be above the ankles with the hips up (forming a tabletop from the neck to the knees). Rest both arms on the side of the ball, with the hands a few inches off the floor (to catch yourself if you start to fall). Slowly straighten one leg at the knee and hold for 8 seconds. Your goal is to do this without the help of your hands on the floor. This is challenging! Repeat on the other leg.

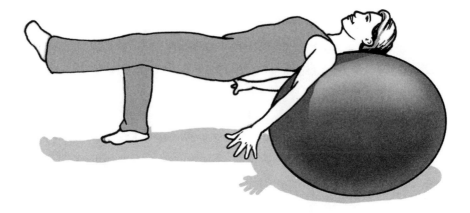

Stretching

The purpose of stretching is to increase the range of motion around the joints by passively moving the joints and muscles beyond their resting range or length. I recommend a weekly stretch or yoga class to improve your flexibility. I have provided a few important stretches that promote good posture, prevent injuries and lower-back pain while increasing mobility in particular areas that tend to shorten with age. Hold all stretches for 1 minute.

Stretching ● beginner and intermediate
Standing Chest Stretch

Stand sideways with your right shoulder to the wall and your left shoulder toward the center of the room. Place your right hand and forearm flat on the wall behind your body and higher than your head. Keep the right elbow bent (at the same height as the shoulder) and turn away from the wall until you feel the stretch in the chest. Repeat with the other arm.

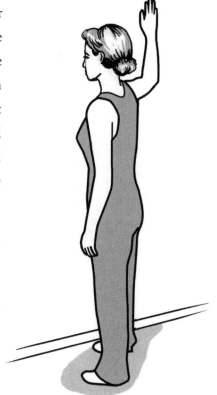

Stretching • beginner and intermediate
Quad and Hip Flexor Stretch

Lie on your side with the bottom arm extended along the floor, above the head, with the head resting flat upon it. Bend the top leg back at the knee and hold with the top hand. Try to grab the foot at the ankle, not the toes. In this position, tuck the buttocks under and press the top hip forward during the stretch. You should feel this up the front of the thigh and at the front of the hip.

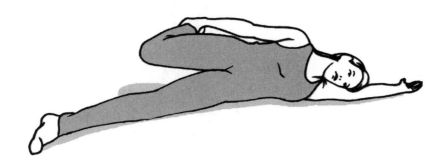

Stretching • beginner and intermediate
Hamstring Stretch

You will need a towel for this stretch. Lie flat on your back with one knee bent up and the other straight up in the air. Wrap the towel around the extended foot and use it to pull the leg towards the chest. Keep the back flat on the floor with the head back also. You should feel this stretch in the belly of the back of the thigh, not behind the knee. Bend the knee slightly to feel the stretch behind the thigh.

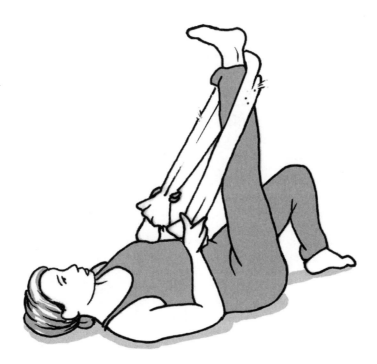

Stretching ••• advanced
Spine and Abdominal Stretch

This is an advanced stretch that should be done with caution and progressed to slowly, over time. Start by sitting on the ball and walk the feet out, letting the ball roll up the spine, and leaning back until the ball is at the middle of the spine (halfway up). Lie back over the ball, letting the head relax back also. Let the spine take the form of the ball and slowly bring the arms up over the head and reach them to the floor. You do not have to go to this level all at once! Take it slow and relax on the ball. If you are tense, you will strain the very muscles that you are trying to stretch.

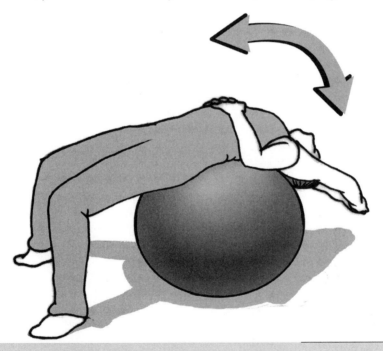

An untrained person who participates in an optimal resistance-training program can increase muscular strength by 30 percent during the first 6–8 weeks of training.

Eight

Functional Fitness
for Every Move

In an aging population, functional training will enhance quality of life through improved confidence, agility and performance in sports and daily living. This in turn will help assure that their later years will be some of the best years of their life.

—Louis J. Stack, owner of Fitter International

Functional fitness is exercise that integrates strength, agility, endurance and flexibility, preparing the body to cope with the physical demands of everyday activities. These activities include getting out of bed, climbing stairs, lifting objects, and bending over and standing back up. They also include unplanned, challenging movements that your body sometimes needs to do, like running to catch a bus, shoveling the driveway, lifting or carrying a heavy object, or regaining balance after your steadiness has been disrupted.

Many of us take these movements or activities for granted, but you will notice that the ease with which you perform them decreases as you age. Functional fitness exercises prepare your body to perform these movements with ease. They also work to prevent the injuries or discomfort associated with doing movements with which your body is not comfortable. For example, suppose you are able to bicep-curl 20 lb. for 15 reps. This means that your biceps are very strong doing that movement. Ask yourself, "What daily activities require me to be good at that very movement?" You may need bicep strength to lift groceries out of the trunk of your car, but you need it in conjunction with lower-back and shoulder strength, hamstring flexibility and overall balance and stability. Functional fitness—integrated movement—helps train your body for the physical demands of everyday life.

Functional Fitness and Aging

When we were younger, the motivation to exercise was frequently based on esthetics. Most of us aspire to a lean, strong, fit-looking body, no matter how old we are. However, something happens as we age: our joints ache in the morning when we rise, our ability to complete simple physical tasks is challenged and we suffer from more chronic aches and pains. The following physiological changes in an aging body directly affect functional fitness.

Range of motion at the joints decreases as movements that challenge that range are no longer done. If you participate in stretching exercises, you continually increase range of motion at your joints when you stretch and hold your muscles past their normal resting length. If you don't stretch on a regular basis, then over time your muscles have shortened, limiting the range of motion at the joints.

Muscular strength decreases as activity levels that challenge the muscles diminish. As we age, our activity level and participation in intense exercise and sport decline. Muscles must be continually challenged to get stronger to support the body and handle movements that are needed to function.

The quality of eyesight is compromised as we age. Your vision is one of a few very important devices that process information about the body's position in space. One's ability to maintain balance depends largely on the quality of vision. Poor balance contributes to falls and, more importantly, lack of confidence in movements. This lack of confidence results in a decrease in physical activity.

Mobility and response time decrease. Although decline in mobility and response time can contribute to accidental injuries often resulting in further immobility, it is the decrease in quality of daily life that is the saddest part of this physiological change. Lack of mobility and slow response time make the simple pleasure of going for a walk difficult and often painful.

Because of these physiological changes, the motivation to exercise comes from a very different place than it did when we were younger. As we age, we are motivated to exercise because we want to be able to maintain and enjoy an active and independent lifestyle. Functional fitness will help us accomplish this goal. It also plays a part in preventing falls that result in bone breaks or fractures because it integrates balance and strength, which assist in stability and confidence in movement.

As stated at the beginning of this chapter, functional fitness integrates movements that require strength, agility, balance, endurance and flexibility. These movements require the activation of postural and stabilizer/neutralizer muscles that are often called core muscles. Functional exercises involve usable movement by training the body for everyday living and simply mimicking the very movements that give you trouble. For example, the sit-stand exercise that has you rising from a chair to a standing position then sitting back down, repeatedly, without the use of the hands, is a functional exercise. It strengthens the quadriceps and hip flexors, maintains center of gravity and improves agility and balance. In practical terms, it helps you get in and out of chairs and cars with greater ease. Functional exercises also improve postural alignment while challenging motor control and balance.

Which Functional Exercises Do I Need?

To decide which functional fitness exercises your body requires, consult your physiotherapist or personal trainer. These professionals are able to examine your movements and assess their individual weaknesses or strengths. They can determine by a person's movements that:

- A particular foot or side is being favored
- Range of motion of a particular joint is limited
- Some specific movements are performed with pain and difficulty
- Specific sites on the body are lacking strength

This does not mean that you can't examine these things yourself and change them. Ask yourself the following questions:

- What makes me sore or ache on a regular basis (determine particular movements)?
- When I walk, how long is my stride (approximately 12 inches or 24)?
- What movements or activities make me nervous while performing them?

- What movements make me feel unsteady?
- What movements do I have difficulty performing?

There are no right answers to these questions. They are designed to make you aware of the physical weaknesses that will only worsen with age, so that you can make changes now. As you move about your day, try to pay attention to the way you move, which activities are difficult and which activities have become harder to do over the past few years. If you examine the ways in which your muscles are required to function in your daily life, you can create a program that will strengthen your body to meet these demands. Do you need to hold on to stable things for balance on a regular basis or do you find it difficult to get in and out of a chair or car? If the answer is yes, these are signs of functional deterioration, but don't despair! After recognizing your weaknesses, you can improve your functional fitness with exercise.

Slower reflexes and decreased strength, combined with loss of eyesight and depth perception, all contribute to a diminished sense of equilibrium.

Incorporating Functional Exercises into Your Program

This is the easy part. Once you have determined the parts of your body or movements you need to work on, you simply need to perform exercises that mimic those movements. In other words, you have to repeatedly practice the very movements that give you trouble. With constant repetition of the movement, the body will strengthen, old neurological patterns will awaken, and confidence in these movements will increase.

With many years of training in this field, I have been able to determine some of the most common movements that deteriorate with age. The following exercises will help you to make these movements easier to perform. Feel free to customize them to your individual needs.

Trouble getting out of a chair, couch or car

Practise getting in and out of a fairly high chair, without using your hands, 10 to 12 times in a row. Progress to a lower chair and then a low couch. Always do 10 to 12 reps to build up strength and increase confidence.

Short stride length (gait)

Walk along a hallway using big, exaggerated steps. Make sure your heel strikes the ground first and you stay tall during the long stride. Try 10 steps in a row, then turn and do the same the other way. Do this 10 times, trying to lengthen your steps each time.

Trouble stepping down off a bus or a high step

Stand on the bottom stair in your home and hold on to the wall or railing beside you. Stand on the left foot at the edge of the step, facing down the stairs, and lower the right foot to the floor below without actually putting it down. Bring the right foot back up and rest it beside the left foot on the step. Repeat the exercise on the same foot 10 times before changing to the other. Make sure the foot is lowered by bending the supporting knee, not the back! Progress by trying this exercise without holding on to anything.

When incorporating functional exercises into your program, adopt the thinking of "Train the movement, not the muscle" and you will be able to create effective exercises for your own needs.

You have now figured out how to incorporate functional exercises into your program. Take the movement that challenges you and perform it in a safe, supported environment. Remember to repeat the movement a number of times.

I am certain that these exercises will assist and improve your strength, agility, balance, endurance and flexibility, and that they will boost your confidence. Do not underestimate how important functional training is to the maintenance of an independent and active lifestyle.

The Bare Bones

- Functional fitness refers to an individual's ability to physically cope with the demands of everyday activities.

- Functional fitness exercises work to prevent injuries while they prepare the body to respond and perform daily tasks with ease. They do this by integrating movements that challenge motor functions, muscular strength, balance and range of motion.

- Functional fitness is especially important for older people because age-related physical changes can be slowed or stopped with functional exercises. These changes are: decreased range of motion at the joints, decreased muscular strength, compromised vision and decreased mobility and response time.

- To add functional exercises to your workout regime, analyze the movements you have difficulty doing and then mimic them repetitively in a controlled environment.

Appendix 1

Movements to Avoid

You should avoid the following three movements if you have—or suspect you have—severe bone loss:

Sudden twisting from the spine (especially while carrying any weight): For example, getting up and out of a car; lifting groceries from the side door of a car.

Suggested correction: Turn the full body—with shoulders and knees in alignment—and place feet firmly on ground before standing, or getting up out of a car. *Always* avoid twisting from the back or waist.

Reaching above shoulder-height: For example, stretching to reach an item on a high shelf.

Suggested correction: Move necessary items to lower storage spaces or—in cases where this is not possible—use a solid stool or stepladder to reach items.

Unsupported forward bending of the spine: For example, bending forward (from the waist) to pick something up.

Suggested correction: Bend from the knees, keeping the waist and back straight, to bring your arms and hands down to the item on the floor.

Appendix 2

Getting "On the Ball":
Safety Tips for Using a Stability Ball

by Phil Delaire, Manager of Fitness and High Performance,
Granite Club (Toronto)

The Swiss or "stability" ball is finally becoming a popular fitness tool in North America. These big, brightly colored inflatable balls represent one of the most important pieces of fitness equipment—beside running shoes—that has come onto the market in a long time.

While relatively new to the United States, stability balls have been used for decades by physical therapists in Europe for rehabilitation and fitness. They are great tools for developing mobilization, coordination, posture, strength and balance. The Swiss ball has even entered the delivery room. During pregnancy, labor and the post-natal period, mothers can perform a wide variety of beneficial exercises.

As with any piece of exercise equipment, a number of equipment guidelines and safety precautions should be kept in mind, including the following.

Size

The correct size of ball you should use is dependent upon your height:

Under 5'2" use a 45 cm ball   5'9"– 6'2" use a 65 cm ball

5'2"– 5'8" use a 55 cm ball   Over 6'3" use a 75 cm ball

Note that when you are sitting on the fully inflated ball your thighs should be parallel to the floor.

Durability

I strongly recommend purchasing a Dura-Ball Swiss Ball. They are anti-burst balls that are much stronger than most. They can be purchased at many fitness stores or ordered from the following distributor:

In U.S.A.: Chek Institute **www.chekinstitute.com** 1-800-552-8789

Inflation

Many companies suggest that you initially inflate a new stability ball to only 80 percent capacity. Leave it underinflated (and do not use it) for 24 hours, then fully inflate it.

It is often difficult to tell if your ball is inflated to the optimum level. The best way to check inflation is to get a ruler and measure the ball from the floor to the top of the ball. The height recorded should match the size of the ball you bought.

Safe Use

When using a stability ball, it is essential that you have a clear space in which to do your exercises so that you won't hit anything around you if you lose your balance. To help prevent uneasiness or falling, practice sitting on the ball and balancing on it in a variety of positions. Make sure you feel comfortable with the ball before you add weight or movement to your exercises.

When lying with your head and upper torso on the ball (see page 185, for example), be sure your *shoulders* are resting solidly on the center of the ball. When attempting exercises in this position, many people place their heads on the center of the ball, which puts undue stress on the neck and encourages poor posture. Ensure that your hips are at the same height as your shoulders and that your knees are bent at a 90 degree angle. Your body, from the shoulders to the knees, should be flat like a tabletop.

Appendix 3
More Bone-Building Exercise Options

Suggestions for Additional Physical Activities

Physical activity of any kind, performed regularly, will help to improve your overall health. But if you are concerned about maintaining or improving your bone density, you should pursue weight-bearing ("impact") and resistance-training activities. Note that some activities will be more effective than others (for example, high- or medium-impact, and high- or medium-resistance exercises).

Keep your initial level of fitness in mind before you explore a new exercise regime. For an exercise program to work, it must exceed the everyday activities that you already perform. If you have not been exercising at all, then beginning by walking (a low-impact exercise) is a great start. You don't need to jump straight in and join a basketball league. If you already walk regularly, then you might want to try stair-climbing or a medium-impact aerobics class. Use common sense and be sure not to overexert yourself or put fragile bones at risk. Consult the table on the next page for examples of high- to low-impact activities.

WEIGHT-BEARING/IMPACT ACTIVITIES

High-impact:	Skipping
	Dancing (medium/high)
	Basketball
	Volleyball
	Court sports (tennis, squash, racketball)
	Soccer
	Running
Medium-impact:	Jogging
	Stair-climbing
	Badminton (medium/high)
Low-impact:	Walking briskly
	Hiking
	Cross-country skiing
	Bowling/Lawn bowling
	Shuffleboard
	Golf
No impact:	Bicycling
	Swimming

RESISTANCE EXERCISES

Medium to High:	Weight-lifting (with hand-held weights, velcro weights, "homemade" weights using cans or jugs, free weights or machines at a gym)
	Exercises using a resistance band
Low:	Aquatics ("Aqua-Fit"-type exercises in the pool)
	Tai Chi

Appendix 4

Progression Training: Adjusting Your Workout Schedule for Maximum Benefit

by Phil Delaire, Manager of Fitness and High Performance, Granite Club (Toronto)

The importance of *progression* in exercise cannot be overemphasized. It is essential that you constantly find new ways of placing stresses on your body. I know some people who have not changed their exercise program in years. Despite the trainer's urgings for change, these people come to the gym at the same time each day, do the same warm-up, complete the same cardiovascular work, the same weight workout, and then do the same stretches to finish up their program. I'm just glad they don't wear the same clothing every day!

It is a simple fact: The more fit you become, the more you need to do in order to stimulate your muscles. If you do the same workout day after day after day—no matter how good it is—your body will eventually stop feeling the benefits.

You can adjust your workout program in three major ways to make sure you keep progressing: in frequency, duration, and intensity.

Frequency

Most people workout anywhere from 2 to 6 times a week.

For Aerobic Exercise

For a change, add another aerobic component to your exercise routine. If you normally go for a brisk walk on Monday, Wednesday and Friday, then switch it up and go Sunday, Tuesday, Thursday. And then if you feel able, add an extra session on Friday. Just this simple switch of days will give your nervous system enough change to make a difference. Adding another workout is an added bonus. Another option is to change the mode you usually choose. Instead of walking, go for a light jog or try the Stairmaster.

For Weight Training

Use the same advice as applied to aerobic exercises: switch the days you normally do weight workouts. However, make sure you don't weight train on consecutive days—be sure to give yourself enough rest between sessions. Usually 48 hours is sufficient.

Duration

For most people, the duration of an average workout is 20 to 60 minutes.

For Aerobic Exercise

If you usually exercise for 20 minutes at a time, then add 10 minutes to one of your workouts in a week. The next week, add another 10 minutes to another one of your workouts (gradually increasing the average time for each workout session). Continue to gradually build like this.

For Weight Training

Most people attempt 8 to 12 repetitions (one set) twice in a workout. If you consistently do this, your body will become accustomed to these two sets. As you progress, add another set, bringing the total number to three. You should never exceed 30 sets total of all exercises in a workout (i.e., three sets each of ten exercises). You should strive to keep it to a total of 25 to 30 sets.

Intensity

For Aerobic Exercise

If you gradually increased your workout time by adding 10 minutes to your aerobic workout each week, by the end of the year you would be doing 2 hours' worth of aerobic exercise each day—and you would be exhausted! Obviously, we don't want you to do that much. Another way you can progress in your program is to increase the intensity with which you approach your workout. The easiest way to do this is to increase the pace you are walking or the level on the bike or Stairmaster that you are using. Alternatively, you can increase the intensity of your workout for a short period of time—5 minutes for example—and then take the exercise back down to your normal intensity. You can do this once in a workout or several times throughout a workout (sometimes referred to as *interval training*). For example, when walking, you could walk for 15 minutes and then jog for 5 minutes, and then repeat. If you are jogging, you could jog for 10 minutes, run hard for 2 minutes, and then repeat.

For Weight Training

If you can manage 12 repetitions in any exercise comfortably, and feel you could do 15 repetitions, then increase the weight 2½ to 5 lbs. If you don't have access to heavier weights, then simply slow down the tempo of your repetitions. If it usually takes you 2 or 3 seconds to finish one repetition, then slow down so that it takes you 4 or 5 seconds. This will have a dramatic effect, and make your workout a little tougher.

Remember: In a workout you have to do more than your body is accustomed to doing, or there will be very little benefit. If you are going to put in the time and effort, make sure you get the results!

Appendix 5
Osteoporosis Resources

Osteoporosis Organizations

International Osteoporosis Foundation
71 Cours Albert Thomas
F-69003 Lyon, France
Tel: +33 472 914177
Fax: +33 472 369052
e-mail: osteofound@net.asi.fr
website: www.ostefound.org

National Osteoporosis Foundation
1232 22nd Street NW
Washington, D.C. 20037-1292
Tel: (202) 223-2226
Fax: (202) 223-2237
website: www.nof.org

Exercise and Nutrition Resources

American Council on Exercise (ACE)
5820 Oberlin Drive, Suite 102
San Diego, California 92121-3787
Tel: (858) 535-8227
Fax: (858) 535-1778
website: www.acefitness.org

Center for Nutrition Policy and Promotion, USDA
1120 20th Street NW, Suite 200
Washington, DC 20036
website: www.usda.gov/cnpp

International Dance and Exercise Association (IDEA)
6190 Cornerstone Court. E, Suite 204
San Diego, California 92121-3773
Tel: 800-999-IDEA or (858) 535-8979
Fax: (858) 535-8234
website: www.IDEAfit.com

Books

Exercise at Menopause: A Critical Difference
Margaret Burghardt, MD
Medscape Women's Health, 1998
website: www.medscape.com

Strong Women, Strong Bones
Miriam E. Nelson with Sarah Wernick
G.P. Putnam's Sons, 1999, New York,

Osteoporosis: How to Make Your Bones Last a Lifetime
Wanda S. Lyon and Cynthia E. Sutton
Tribune Publishing, 1993, Orlando, Florida

The Osteoporosis Handbook
(2nd Edition)
Sydney Lou Bonnick
Taylor Publishing, 1997, New York

Calcium "Plus" Workbook for Healthy Bodies
Evelyn P. Whitelock
Keats Publishing, 1988, Illinois

End Notes

1 Understanding Osteoporosis

1. National Osteoporosis Foundation "Fast Facts on Osteoporosis" www.nof.org
2. Romanes, G.J. *Cunningham's Textbook of Anatomy* (London: Oxford University Press, 1972).
3. Kanis, J. *Osteoporosis* (London: Blackwell Science, 1997).
4. Brands, B. *Management of Alcohol, Tobacco and other Drug Problems* (Toronto: Centre for Addiction and Mental Health, 2000).
5. Pappioannou, A., et al. "Mortality, independence in living and re-fracture, one year following hip fracture in Canadians." *Journal of the Society of Obstetrics and Gynecology of Canada* 22(8) (2000):591–597.
6. Schiller, P.C., et al. "Inhibition of gap junctional communication induces the trans-differentiation of human osteoblastic cells to an adipocytic phenotype in culture." *Journal of Bone and Mineral Research* 15 (Suppl 1) (2000):S139.
7. Eisman, J.A., et al. "Genetics of osteoporosis and vitamin D receptor alleles." *Calcified Tissue International* 56 (Suppl 1) (1995):S48–S49.
8. Lyles, K.W., et al. "Vertebral number and site correlation with impairments." American Geriatric Society Annual Meeting, May 6–10, 1998:167, P248.
9. Dempster, D. "The contribution of trabecular architecture to cancellous bone quality." *Journal of Bone and Mineral Research* 15 (2000):20–23.
10. World Health Organization. "Assessment of fracture risk and its application to screening for postmenopausal osteoporosis." No. 843 of Technical Reports Series (Geneva: The Organization, 1994).

2 The Bone Boosters: Calcium and Vitamin D

1. Beck, L. *Managing Menopause with Diet, Vitamins and Herbs* (Toronto: Prentice Hall Canada, 2000), 116.
2. Heaney, R.P., McCarron, D.A., Dawson-Hughes, B., et al. "Dietary Changes Favorably Affect Bone Remodeling in Older Adults." *Journal of the American Dietetic Association* 99(10) (Oct. 1999):1228–1233.
3. "Calcium for postmenopausal osteoporosis." *The Medical Letter* 24(623) (1982):105–106.
4. Heaney, R.P., et al. "Absorption of calcium as the carbonate and citrate salts, with some observation in method." *Osteoporosis International* 9 (1999):19–23.
5. Glerup, H., Mikkelsen, K., Poulsen, L., et al. "Commonly recommended daily

intake of vitamin D is not sufficient if sunlight exposure is limited." *Journal of Internal Medicine* 247(2) (February 2000):260–268 Abstract.

6. Sahota, O. "Osteoporosis and the role of calcium-vitamin D deficiency, vitamin D insufficiency and vitamin D sufficiency." *Age and Aging* 29 (2000):301–304.

7. *Osteoporosis Bulletin for Physicians* 2 (4) (May 1994).

8. Chapuy, M.C., et al. "Vitamin D_3 and calcium prevent hip fractures in elderly women." *New England Journal of Medicine* 327 (1992):1637.

3 More Bone Boosters: Other Nutritional Strategies

1. Ewan, G. "Let's put calcium bioavailability in perspective." Editorial. *Nutrition Quarterly* 18(1) (1984).

2. Cohen, L., and Kitzes, R. "Infrared spectroscopy and magnesium content of bone mineral in osteoporotic women." *Israel Journal of Medical Science* 17 (1981):1123–1125.

3. Tucker, K.L., Hannan, M.T., Chen, H., et al. "Potassium, magnesium, and fruit and vegetable intakes are associated with greater bone mineral density in elderly men and women." *American Journal of Clinical Nutrition* 69(4) (April 1999):727–736.

4. Hodges, D. "Do soft drinks soften bones?" The Nutrition Factor, *The Medical Post*, July 4, 2000.

5. Nelson, M.E. *Strong Bones* (New York: G.P. Putman's Sons, 1999), 111.

6. Murray, M.T. *Encyclopedia of Nutritional Supplements* (Rocklin, California: Prima Health, Prima Publishing,1996).

7. Neilson, E.H., et al. "Effect of dietary boron on mineral. estrogen, and testosterone metabolism in postmenopausal women." *FASEB Journal* 1 (1987):394–397.

4 Drug Strategies to Prevent and Treat Osteoporosis

1. Graham, J., et al. "Time out for perimenopause." *Canadian Journal of Diagnosis* 17(10) (2000):75–87.

2. Scientific Advisory Board, Osteoporosis Society of Canada. "Clinical practice guidelines for the diagnosis and management of osteoporosis." *Canadian Medical Association Journal* 155(8) (1996):1113–1133.

3. The Working Group for the PEPI Trial. "Effects of estrogen/progestin regimes in postmenopausal women: the Postmenopausal Estrogen/Progestin Interventions (PEPI) Trial." *Journal of the American Medical Association (JAMA)* 273 (1995):199–208.

4. Hulley, S., et al. "Randomized trial of estrogen plus progestin for secondary prevention of coronary heart disease in postmenopausal women. Heart and Estrogen/Progestin Replacement Study (HERS) Research Group." *Journal of the American Medical* Association *(JAMA)* 280 (1998):605–613.

5. Wilson, W. "Should women with coronary disease be prescribed hormone replacement therapy?" *Chronical of Cardiovascular and Internal Medicine* 12 (1999):6.

6. Ettinger, B., et al. "Reduction of vertebral fracture risk in postmenopausal women with osteoporosis treated with raloxifene." *Journal of the American Medical Association (JAMA)* 282 (1999):637–645.

7. Chestnut, C.H., et al. "A randomized trial of nasal spray salmon calcitonin in post-menopausal women with established osteoporosis: The Prevent Recurrence of Osteoporotic Fractures Study." *American Journal of Medicine* 109 (2000):267–276; Halkin, V., et al. "Efficacy and tolerability of calcitonin in the prevention and treatment of osteoporosis." *BioDrugs* 10(4) (1998):295–300.

8. Black, D.M., et al. "Randomized trial of effect of alendronate on risk of fracture in women with existing vertebral fractures." Lancet 348 (1996):1535–1541; Cummings, S.R., et al. "Effect of alendronate on risk of fracture on women with low bone density, but without vertebral fractures." *Journal of the American Medical Association (JAMA)* 280(24) (1998):2077–2082; Harris, S.T., et al. "Effects of risedronate treatment on vertebral and non-vertebral fractures with post-menopausal osteoporosis." *Journal of the American Medical Association (JAMA)* 282(14) (1999):1344–1352.

5 Exercise: The Magic Cure?

1. Morganti, C.M., Nelson, M.E., Fiatarone, M.A., et al. "Strength improvements with 1 yr. of progressive resistance training in older women." *Medicine and Science in Sports and Exercise* 27(6) (1995):906–912.

2. Huddleston, A.L., Rockwell, D., Kuland, D.N., et al. "Bone mass in lifetime tennis players." *Journal of the American Medical Association (JAMA)* 244 (1980):1107–1109.

3. Notellovitz, M., and Martin, D. "Effects of aerobic exercise on bone mineral density of postmenopausal women." *Medicine and Science in Sports and Exercise* 25 (Supp 5) (1993):S199.

4. Guiton, A.C. *Human Physiology and Mechanisms of Disease*, 5th ed. (London: W.B. Saunders Company), 644–645.

5. Kontulainen, S., Kannus, P., Haapasalo, H., et al. "Changes in bone mineral content with decreased training in competitive young adult tennis players and

controls: a prospective 4-yr follow-up." Bone Research Group, *Finland Medicine and Science in Sports and Exercise* 5 (May 1999):31.

6. Heinon, A., et al. "Bone Mineral Density in Female Athletes Representing Sports with Different Loading Characteristics of the Skeleton." *Bone* 3 (September 1995):197–203.

7. Dook, J.E., James, C., Henderson, N.K., and Price, R.I. "Exercise and Bone Mineral Density in Mature Female Athletes." *Medicine and Science in Sports and Exercise* 29(3) (March 1997):291–296.

8. Tinetti, M.E., et al. "A Multifactorial Intervention to Reduce the Risk of Falling Among Elderly People Living in the Community." *New England Journal of Medicine* 13 (September 1994):821–829.

9. Myers, A.H., Young, Y., and Langlois, J.A. "Prevention of Falls in the Elderly." *Bone* 1 (January 1996):87S–101S.

10. Neporent, L. "Balance Drills, for the Sake of Safety." *New York Times Sci* (January 1999).

11. Drinkwater, B.L., Bruemner, B., and Chesnut, C.H. "Menstrual history as a determinant of current bone density in young adults." *Journal of the American Medical Association (JAMA)* 263(4) (January 1990):545–548.

12. Fruth, S.J., and Worrell, T.M. "Factors associated with menstrual irregularities and decreased bone mineral density in female athletes." *Journal of Orthopedic Sports and Physical Therapy* 22(1) (July 1995):26–38.

Glossary

aerobic activities
any exercises during which the body utilizes oxygen

age-related bone loss
bone loss caused by an imbalance between the formation (building) and resorption (taking away) of bone caused by aging

amenorrhea
absence or abnormal stoppage of menstrual cycles

anterior deltoid
muscle group on the front of the shoulders

antioxidant
a substance that inhibits another substance from reacting chemically with oxygen, thus preventing tissue damage

apoptosis
programmed or planned cell death

balance-stability
an equilibrium or steadiness of the body, important in the prevention of falls

biceps
the largest muscle on the front of the arm

bioavailability
the degree to which a drug or substance becomes available to the target tissue after administration

biochemical markers
the byproducts of the body's chemistry that are found in the blood

bisphosphonates
a family of drugs used to treat osteoporosis

bone density
the amount of bone in a certain volume

bone markers
the byproducts of bone remodeling found in the blood

bone mass
the amount of bone

bone mineral density test (BMD)
the test used to measure bone mass and density

bone scan
a special bone X-ray that detects fractures, arthritis, cancer in the bone and some other bone diseases

boron
a trace mineral found in the body in very small amounts, but necessary for bone health

breast self-examination (BSE)
a special method of examining your breasts yourself to detect breast lumps

calcitonin
a hormone made by the thyroid gland that lowers blood calcium level and decreases bone resorption or loss

calcium
a chemical element that is essential for the body, particularly for the bones

calcium absorption
the process by which calcium is absorbed from the intestine into the blood

calcium salts
a compound of calcium and another substance that enables calcium to move in the body, i.e., calcium carbonate, calcium citrate

calf
the back part of the leg below the knee

cardiorespiratory system
the body system that includes the heart, arteries, veins and lungs

cholecalciferol
a form of vitamin D

contraindication
something that would cause a particular medication or course of treatment to be inappropriate

cortex (bone)
the dense outer shell of bone

dowager's hump
a hump in the upper back, usually caused by fracturing of the vertebrae or back bones; see *kyphosis*

effort level
a subjective measurement of physical exertion related to exercise

electrolyte
a mineral salt that carries a charge and is always found paired with another electrolyte of opposite charge

endometrium
the lining of the uterus

estrogen
female sex hormone produced by the ovaries and responsible for breast development and sexual maturation of girls

estrogen replacement therapy (ERT)
replacement of estrogen with medication after menopause

exercise band
a long, stretchy, rubber ribbon used for exercise

exercise log
a written record of your exercise program

fitness
the health of the cardiorespiratory system, muscular strength, muscular endurance and flexibility

flexibility
the range of motion available around a joint

formation (bone)
production of new bone by the osteoblasts

functional fitness
the ability to physically cope with demands of everyday activities

hamstrings
muscles on the back of the thigh behind the knee

high density lipoprotein (HDL)
a combination of fat and protein that is measured in the blood that helps your doctor assess risk for heart attack or stroke; also called "good" cholesterol

hormone replacement therapy (HRT)
replacement of estrogen and progesterone with medication after menopause

hot flashes
a menopausal symptom of feeling hot and sweaty, accompanied by reddening of the skin, particularly the face

hysterectomy
surgical removal of the womb (uterus)

intensity [exercise]
refers to "how hard" the body is working during exercise

insoluble fiber
found in cereals; increases fecal bulk and frequency

isoflavones
a plant estrogen found in soy products that mimics estrogen

kyphosis
a hump in the upper back usually caused by fracturing of the vertebrae or back bones; also known as *dowager's hump*

lactose
the sugar found in milk, made up of glucose and galactose

lactose intolerance
the inability to digest lactose, the sugar found in milk

lats
largest muscle group across the back

low density lipoprotein (LDL)
carries cholesterol through the bloodstream; high levels increase risk of heart disease; also called the "bad" cholesterol

magnesium
a chemical element found in the body, involved in many of the body's enzyme reactions and essential for good bone health

mammogram
an X-ray of the breast used to detect breast cancer

mechanical loading
causing the bone to work against a load; when a joint is moved to a different position, the muscles and ligaments either push or pull on the bone, whose internal structures resist all such forces

medial deltoid
middle shoulder muscles

menopause
twelve months without a menstrual period

muscular endurance
the body's ability to maintain a physical activity while resisting muscular fatigue

muscular strength
the body's ability to exert force against a resistance during muscular contraction

NTx (N-teleopeptide cross links)
a byproduct of bone resorption found in the blood and urine

osteoblasts
bone-building cells taking part in bone formation

osteoclasts
bone-removal cells taking part in bone resorption

osteocalcin
a byproduct of bone formation or building found in the blood

osteocytes
resting osteoblasts found in bone that send messages through the bone

osteoid
a soft, protein-containing material that becomes hardened with calcium and forms into strong, new healthy bone

osteoporosis
a disease in which the bones become increasingly porous, brittle and prone to fracture

osteopenia
thin bones, but not as thin and weak as osteoporotic bones

parathyroid hormone
a regulator of bone, secreted by the parathyroid gland

peak bone mass
the maximum bone density and strength that a person can attain

phytic acid
found in the bran of whole grains; likely to interfere with calcium absorption; binds to a variety of minerals, including calcium, to form insoluble salts that are excreted by the body as waste

phytoestrogens
estrogens made from plants, such as yams or soy

posterior deltoid
muscles found at the back of the shoulder

postmenopausal osteoporosis
at menopause, estrogen deprivation causes rapid bone loss, particularly for the first ten years after menopause, leading to this condition

progesterone
a female sex hormone made in the ovaries and placenta

progestin
a female sex hormone made in the ovaries and placenta

progression
advancement and development that leads to improvement in the performance of a physical activity

quadriceps
muscles located in the front of the thigh

reflex
a physical response to a stimulus

remodeling
the process of continual formation and resorption in bones

reps (repetitions)
the number of times you complete an exercise movement from start to finish, continuously

resistance
the amount of weight or load placed upon a specific muscle group

resistance training
an exercise that stresses the muscles by moving a weight against gravity; involves the contraction or shortening of the muscle fiber

resorption
the removal of bone

rhomboids
muscles between the shoulder blades

rotator cuff
rotational muscles of the shoulder

secondary osteoporosis
osteoporosis caused by any medical problem other than aging and menopause

selective estrogen receptor modulators (SERMs)
a class of drugs with some estrogenlike and some non-estrogenlike properties

sets
the number of groups of repetitions

soluble fiber
found in fruit, beans, food gums and oats; binds and removes "bad" cholesterol from the body

stability ball
a soft, plastic ball filled with air, used for exercise; also known as a "Swiss" ball

standard deviation (SD)
the difference between your BMD (bone mineral density) and that of a healthy young adult

tamoxifen
the first SERM, now mainly used to treat breast cancer

trabecular bone
the internal supporting structure or struts of the bone

triceps
back upper arm muscle

U.S. Recommended Daily Allowance (RDA)
the amount of a nutrient recommended for daily intake, also known as Reference Daily Intake

vitamin D
the sunshine vitamin that helps to absorb calcium from the intestine

vitamin D deficiency
an insufficient amount of vitamin D causing low absorption of calcium from the intestine, thus necessitating the use of the body's stored bone calcium

warm-up
an activity that brings blood to the muscle groups and lubricates the joints, preparing them for exercise

weight-bearing exercises
exercises that are done while supporting your own body weight

Index